T0146021

Narrative Matters

Health Affairs

Narrative Matters

Writing to Change the Health Care System

SECOND EDITION

Edited by Jessica Bylander
Senior Editor, *Health Affairs*

Foreword by Abraham Verghese, MD

Johns Hopkins University Press / Baltimore

This book is dedicated to Fitzhugh Mullan, 1942–2019.

© 2020 Project HOPE–The People-to-People Health Foundation, Inc.
Foreword copyright © 2019 by Abraham Verghese. All rights reserved. Reprinted
by arrangement with Mary Evans Inc.
All rights reserved. Published 2020
Printed in the United States of America on acid-free paper
9 8 7 6 5 4 3 2 1

This book was published in a first edition as *Narrative Matters: The Power
of the Personal Essay in Health Policy*, edited by Fitzhugh Mullan, MD, Ellen
Ficklen, and Kyna Rubin (Baltimore: Johns Hopkins University Press, 2006).

Johns Hopkins University Press
2715 North Charles Street
Baltimore, Maryland 21218-4363
www.press.jhu.edu

Library of Congress Cataloging-in-Publication Data

Names: Bylander, Jessica, editor.
Title: Narrative matters : writing to change the health care system /
    edited by Jessica Bylander, senior editor, *Health Affairs*; foreword by
    Abraham Verghese, MD.
Description: Second edition. | Baltimore : Johns Hopkins University Press,
    2020. | Includes index.
Identifiers: LCCN 2019029985 | ISBN 9781421437521 (hardcover) |
    ISBN 9781421437545 (paperback) | ISBN 9781421437552 (ebook)
Subjects: LCSH: Medical policy. | Narrative medicine.
Classification: LCC RA393 .N37 2020 | DDC 362.1—dc23
LC record available at https://lccn.loc.gov/2019029985

A catalog record for this book is available from the British Library.

William Stafford, excerpt from "You Reading This, Be Ready" from *Ask Me:
100 Essential Poems*. Copyright © 1980, 1998 by William Stafford and the
Estate of William Stafford. Reprinted with the permission of The Permissions
Company, LLC on behalf of Graywolf Press, Minneapolis, Minnesota,
www.graywolfpress.org.

*Special discounts are available for bulk purchases of this book. For more
information, please contact Special Sales at specialsales@press.jhu.edu.*

Johns Hopkins University Press uses environmentally friendly book materials,
including recycled text paper that is composed of at least 30 percent post-
consumer waste, whenever possible.

Contents

Foreword

What a treat to write a foreword a second time for a *second* collection of the best essays submitted to the "Narrative Matters" section of *Health Affairs*. The last such volume was over a decade ago. I love seeing how the grand experiment by Fitzhugh Mullan and John Iglehart in adding a new section to the esteemed journal *Health Affairs* has become so established that most readers will assume it has always been there.

When "Narrative Matters" was first conceived, I wondered if it would survive. The very idea of a highly respected medical journal publishing stories that captured poignant human lessons of heartache, joy, and redemption was still new; those of us who wrote such pieces were suspect and we admitted to authorship sheepishly, knowing full well the coin of the realm, particularly in a journal read by those in the C-suite (who often paid my salary), was *data*. When the time came to economize, would this qualitative section of the journal (or in the parlance of undergrads, the "fuzzy" as opposed to the "techy" section) be jettisoned to keep the ship afloat? I find it delightful to see how well it has thrived.

We have come a long way. Story and story seminars and finding your story are all the rage now, the staple of executive coaching seminars and business school retreats within and without the health care enterprise. Thank God for that.

Kant's *Critique of Pure Reason* opens famously with the words, "That all our knowledge begins with experience there can be no doubt." In medicine, for the longest time it seemed true that "experience" meant the quantified experience with raw numbers valued over the subjective experience of care; what the doctor or patient felt was less important than what could be measured. But "Narrative Matters" drew a line in the sand. It said that in the world of health care, in the $3 trillion trough at which we all feed and where reimbursement drives practice, stories matter. Stories change our lives.

If you don't believe stories have power, think of Harriet Beecher Stowe's *Uncle Tom's Cabin*: that story is what ended slavery in America. It wasn't a president, a congress, or an army but a change in public sentiment triggered by that tale that ended slavery. The book *The Citadel*, by A. J. Cronin, is thought to be responsible for the birth of the UK's National Health Service, because the fictional tale of health care conditions in a coal-mining region reflected a shocking reality and rallied the public. The stories of Ryan White and Magic Johnson changed the tenor of conversations around AIDS. From the Tuskegee story of rogue research in syphilis to the story of Henrietta Lacks, stories shape health care, shape trust. Narrative has always mattered.

The reflective essays found in this volume are the very best of the recent years. Although the editors have put them in categories, the authors surely did not write them with a category in mind. Instead, they wrote because of something that deeply affected them, something they lived through or observed, and you can be sure it was always personal and heartfelt.

And for us, the readers, the effect is striking and uniform: we are moved and we carry away some new understanding, one we would be hard pressed to convey to another except through story. Narrative moves us. It drives us to the kind of insight and realization that William Stafford captures in a few lines from his poem "You Reading This, Be Ready":

> . . . lift this
> new glimpse that you found; carry into evening

all that you want from this day. This interval you spent
reading or hearing this, keep it for life—

What can anyone give you greater than now,
starting here, right in this room, when you turn around?

So, dear reader. Start now. Be ready.

Abraham Verghese, MD, MACP, FRCP (Edin)
Linda R. Meier and Joan F. Lane Provostial Professor
Vice Chair for the Theory and Practice of Medicine
Stanford University

Contributors

Louise Aronson is a professor of geriatrics at the University of California, San Francisco (UCSF), where her roles include medical education and directing UCSF Health Humanities. She is also the author of a short story collection, *A History of the Present Illness* (Bloomsbury, 2013), and the nonfiction *Elderhood: Redefining Aging, Transforming Medicine, Reimagining Life* (Bloomsbury, 2019).

Laura Arrowsmith is a physician, educator, and advocate for the transgender community. She is a contributor to *Transgender and Gender Diverse Persons: A Handbook for Service Providers, Educators, and Families* (Routledge, 2018). She is based in Tulsa, Oklahoma.

Cheryl Bettigole is the director of Get Healthy Philly, the Division of Chronic Disease and Injury Prevention of the Philadelphia Department of Public Health. She is a past president of the National Physicians Alliance in Washington, DC.

Cindy Brach is cochair of the Health Literacy Work Group of the US Department of Health and Human Services and a senior health care researcher at the Agency for Healthcare Research and Quality (AHRQ) in Rockville, Maryland.

GARY EPSTEIN-LUBOW is the medical director of the Center for Memory Health at Hebrew SeniorLife in Boston. He is an associate professor of psychiatry and human behavior, and of medical science, at the Alpert Medical School of Brown University and an associate professor of health services, policy, and practice at the Brown University School of Public Health. He is also a visiting associate professor of psychiatry at Harvard Medical School.

JONATHAN FRIEDLAENDER is an emeritus professor of biological anthropology at Temple University in Philadelphia, Pennsylvania. He has been a patient representative for the Food and Drug Administration in Silver Spring, Maryland. He has held positions at Harvard University, the University of Wisconsin–Madison, and the National Science Foundation.

PATRICIA GABOW is professor emerita at the University of Colorado School of Medicine and former CEO of Denver Health.

KATTI GRAY is a freelance writer, editor, and journalism lecturer who specializes in covering health, criminal justice, and education for a range of national publications.

YASMIN SOKKAR HARKER is a professor and law librarian at the City University of New York School of Law in New York City.

TIMOTHY HOFF is a professor of management, health care systems, and health policy at Northeastern University in Boston, Massachusetts, and a visiting associate fellow at Green-Templeton College and visiting scholar at Saïd Business School, both at the University of Oxford. He is the author of *Next in Line: Lowered Care Expectations in the Age of Retail- and Value-Based Health* (Oxford University Press, 2017) and *Practice under Pressure: Primary Care Physicians and Their Medicine in the Twenty-First Century* (Rutgers University Press, 2009).

CARLA KEIRNS is an assistant professor of history and philosophy of medicine and an assistant professor of internal medicine at the University of Kansas Medical Center in Kansas City, Kansas.

RAYA ELFADEL KHEIRBEK is a professor of medicine and chief of the Palliative Medicine Division at the University of Maryland School of Medicine in Baltimore, Maryland.

KATY B. KOZHIMANNIL is an associate professor in the Division of Health Policy and Management at the University of Minnesota School of Public Health in Minneapolis.

POOJA LAGISETTY is an assistant professor in the Division of General Internal Medicine at the University of Michigan and a research investigator at the Veterans Affairs Ann Arbor Healthcare System.

MARIA MALDONADO is an associate professor of medicine and director of education in cross-cultural and patient-centered communication at the Icahn School of Medicine at Mount Sinai in New York City. She also practices primary care medicine in Yonkers, New York.

MAUREEN A. MAVRINAC is board-certified in family medicine and geriatrics and currently works with vulnerable elderly patients in inner-city Los Angeles.

DIANE E. MEIER is the director of the Center to Advance Palliative Care, a professor in the Department of Geriatrics and Palliative Medicine, and the Catherine Gaisman Professor of Medical Ethics at the Icahn School of Medicine at Mount Sinai in New York City.

DINA KELLER MOSS is the ACTION III lead at the Agency for Healthcare Research and Quality in Rockville, Maryland. ACTION III research supports the development and testing of interventions designed to improve care delivery and the dissemination and implementation of successful care delivery models in diverse care settings.

SIDDHARTHA MUKHERJEE is an assistant professor of medicine at Columbia University in New York City and a cancer physician and researcher. He is the author of *The Emperor of All Maladies: A Biography of Cancer* (Scribner, 2010), which won the 2011 Pulitzer Prize in general nonfiction; *The Laws of Medicine: Field Notes from an Uncertain Science* (Simon & Schuster, 2015); and *The Gene: An Intimate History* (Scribner, 2017).

DONNA JACKSON NAKAZAWA is an award-winning science journalist and the author of *The Angel and the Assassin: The Tiny Brain Cell That Changed the Course of Medicine* (Ballantine, 2019), *Childhood Disrupted* (Atria Books, 2015), *The Last Best Cure* (Avery, 2013), and *The Autoimmune Epidemic* (Touchstone, 2008).

TRAVIS N. RIEDER is the assistant director for education initiatives and a research scholar at the Johns Hopkins Berman Institute of Bioethics in Baltimore, Maryland. He is the author of *In Pain: A Bioethicist's Personal Struggle with Opioids* (HarperCollins, 2019).

AROONSIRI SANGARLANGKARN is lead geriatrician at the HIV Netherlands Australia Thailand Research Collaboration (HIV-NAT) Clinic, Thai Red Cross Society, in Bangkok.

ELAINE SCHATTNER is a writer, patient advocate, and physician who lives in New York City.

JANICE LYNCH SCHUSTER is a poet and artist living in Annapolis, Maryland. She is a coauthor of an award-winning book, *Handbook for Mortals: Guidance for People Facing Serious Illness* (Oxford University Press, second edition, 2011), and a frequent contributor to the *Washington Post*.

MYRICK C. SHINALL is a surgeon and palliative care physician at Vanderbilt University Medical Center in Nashville, Tennessee, where he also works in the Center for Biomedical Ethics and Society.

GAYATHRI SUBRAMANIAN is an assistant professor in the Department of Diagnostic Sciences at Rutgers School of Dental Medicine in Newark, New Jersey.

LOUIS W. SULLIVAN is chair of the Sullivan Alliance to Transform the Health Professions in Washington, DC. He served as Secretary of Health and Human Services from 1989 to 1993 and is the founding dean and president emeritus of Morehouse School of Medicine in Atlanta, Georgia. He is the coauthor of *The Morehouse Mystique: Becoming a Doctor at the Nation's Newest African American Medical School* (with Marybeth Gasman) (Johns Hopkins University Press, 2012) and *Breaking Ground: My Life in Medicine* (with David Chanoff) (University of Georgia Press, 2014).

GAUTHAM K. SURESH is a professor of pediatrics at the Baylor College of Medicine and section head and service chief of neonatology at Texas Children's Hospital, both in Houston, Texas.

ABRAHAM VERGHESE is the Linda R. Meier and Joan F. Lane Provostial Professor and vice chair for the theory and practice of medicine in the Department of Medicine at Stanford University. He is the author of *My Own Country* (Vintage Books, 1994), *The Tennis Partner* (HarperCollins, 1998), and *Cutting for Stone* (Alfred A. Knopf, 2009), as well as short stories and essays.

OTIS WARREN is an associate professor of emergency medicine at the Warren Alpert Medical School, Brown University, in Providence, Rhode Island.

LEANA S. WEN is an emergency physician and public health leader who is on the faculty at George Washington University School of

Medicine and the Johns Hopkins Bloomberg School of Public Health. She is the former president/CEO of the Planned Parenthood Federation of America, and before that served as the Baltimore City Health Commissioner.

CHARLOTTE YEH is chief medical officer for AARP Services Inc., where she works with companies that provide AARP-branded programs to enhance care for older adults.

Introduction

A cancer patient receives treatment and is disease-free, but the anxiety of cancer in the future—fed by new technologies that radically alter the landscape of cancer risk and screening—haunts her. A transgender physician is mocked and mistreated by a health care provider and vows to make the system better for patients like herself. A melanoma survivor struggles to access an unapproved—but clinically promising—drug to treat his disease. A patient receives prescription opioids after a motorcycle accident—and no support from his physicians as he agonizingly weans himself off.

These stories are among those featured in the 32 essays selected for inclusion in this second anthology of essays from the "Narrative Matters" section of *Health Affairs*. (The first such anthology was published in 2006.) The personal experiences with the health care system conveyed in these essays are occasionally infuriating, often indelible, and always instructive. They reflect the mission of this unique section of *Health Affairs*, a section that blends personal narratives with their health policy implications to create *policy narratives* that aim to add much-needed human context to evidence-based health care decision-making. The best "Narrative Matters" essays have a compelling personal story at their core, coupled with a clear call for policy action.

As Fitzhugh Mullan, a professor, physician, and the first editor of "Narrative Matters," wrote in the section's inaugural essay, "Me and the System: The Personal Essay and Health Policy," in 1999, "Health (and health policy) is a quintessentially human realm, and its stories are as vivid and revealing as those from any area of human endeavor. Even as we move to put decision-making in health on a firmer, more quantitative basis, our stories can help to maintain perspective and promote wisdom. That is the mission of 'Narrative Matters.'"

Though the section was considered a bit of an experiment at the time, its place in the journal now feels cemented: "Narrative Matters" celebrated its twentieth year in July 2019, and to date *Health Affairs* has published more than 250 essays in the section—along with some poetry, as well.

That the "Narrative Matters" section survives—and thrives—after 20 years is an indication not only that narrative still matters but also that the health care system still benefits from the essayist's attention. The topics covered in this new volume touch on familiar challenges, such as appropriate end-of-life care, as well as new issues of the day, including opioid use disorders, transgender health care, and the impact of national immigration policies on the practice of medicine.

In the decades since "Narrative Matters" launched, the field of medical and health narratives has also seen tremendous growth and diversification. Columbia University's Program in Narrative Medicine, developed by general internist and literary scholar Rita Charon in 2000, has grown in popularity and now features both a master's degree and certification program in narrative medicine. And in 2007, physician and artist Ian Williams created the Graphic Medicine website, which has expanded into a series of graphic novels about health and health care, graphic medicine conferences, and more. Writing and other art forms increasingly provide an outlet for patients, families, clinicians, policy makers, and others invested in health care to make their voices heard in the interest of bettering a system that most would agree does not always serve us as well as it should.

As Charon remarked in her 2018 Jefferson Lecture in the Humanities, the highest honor the federal government bestows for distinguished intellectual achievement in the humanities, "Bridging the chasms between the arts and the sciences, between literature and medicine, quite remarkably, improves the care of the sick."

The 32 essays in this book are organized around themes, including the practice of medicine, medical innovation and research, disparities and discrimination, and aging and end-of-life care. The aim of the essays in this book, and of every essay in the "Narrative Matters" section of *Health Affairs*, is to spark thoughtful conversation and to contribute lived experiences and accounts to sometimes faceless policy debates. For educators in the growing field of medical and health narrative study, the book will inform curricula and stimulate future writing.

The desire is for readers to pull this new collection of "Narrative Matters" essays off the shelf time and again, as the pieces in the volume deserve frequent revisiting. We hope, too, that readers will be encouraged to write and submit content of their own to the section, ensuring that this type of writing about health and health policy endures for decades more.

Narrative Matters

1

The Practice of Medicine

The Importance of Being

Good patient care is found not on a computer screen but in being truly present with patients.

Abraham Verghese

Recently a colleague asked if I would address a small, informal quarterly gathering of hospitalists. We settled on a date, and when she asked me for a title for my remarks, I offered: "Presence."

From the pause on the other end of the line, it was clear she seemed to think there was more to follow—a subtitle perhaps, without which the word seemed to dangle.

"Just 'presence'?"

(I'd been doodling on the paper in front of me, trying it out.)

"Yes," I said. "Presence, period."

On the paper, the period seemed critical. (I'm reminded of the precocious boy-narrator in an Isaac Babel story who says, "No iron can pierce the human heart as icily as a well-placed period.") My period asked me, the reader, to stay with the word—to be present. No subtitle. Just: Presence.

The idea of "presence" had its origins for me in a parking lot not far from my office at Stanford University and near one of my favorite spots on campus, the Rodin Sculpture Garden. In walking past Auguste Rodin's *Gates of Hell*, a massive pair of bronze doors inspired by Dante's *Inferno*, I'm consciously or subconsciously reminded to seize the day. In the past year, I'd watched construction on a unique building in the same vicinity. The signage said it was to be the home for the modern art collection of one family, the Andersons, who were giving the collection to Stanford. From a distance, it looked like a cake box sitting on a narrower and well-lit square pedestal.

Volume 35, Number 10. October 2016.

It occurred to me that the intent of the university and of the Andersons might be that the collection should not only enhance our lives as viewers but specifically enhance our lives as *educators*, even in fields far removed from art history—fields such as my own of internal medicine and infectious diseases. In clinical teaching, I've tried when I can to link art and medicine using such iconic paintings as Luke Fildes's *The Doctor*. But with modern art, with the abstract, it feels challenging to make such a connection. In truth, modern art has always felt a little intimidating to me.

One afternoon shortly after the museum opened, on my way back to my car, I impulsively decided to walk in. It was spring. I felt brave. I imagined the lead up to a punch line: "A physician walks into a modern art museum . . ." After all, this isn't a place where we routinely find ourselves, or if we do, it's not related to work. Personally, I felt my visit *was* related to work and not just by proximity to my place of work: I was here in the true spirit of an educator (so I told myself) trying to climb out of what novelist Walker Percy called the ruts of specialization, the narrow chutes of professional work and our specialized language that can leave us wearing blinders to other forms of knowledge and inquiry.

The building was suffused with natural light. There were no corridors, no rooms that led into rooms, no sense of a labyrinth. Instead it was open—the cake box sans cake. I could and did stroll around the whole thing in 15 minutes. It was much less intimidating than, say, the Louvre, where a tourist popping in for a few hours (after standing in line for a long time) can come away overwhelmed, feeling the mind has been shrunk instead of expanded. And yet the compact space (by museum standards) held a who's who of modern art: Jackson Pollock, Mark Rothko, Willem de Kooning, Wayne Thiebaud, and many more. Iconic names. I had a vague *cognitive* knowledge of that kind of art but no experience. Just as I might know who RuPaul is, or 50 Cent, or Amy Winehouse—but don't ask me to hum a tune.

I was pleased with myself after my visit. Whatever fears I had (about being grilled about my knowledge by docents, or scrutinized by security guards, or finding the art to be opaque and mysterious) were unfounded. The place was inviting and friendly.

From then on, I made it a practice to stop in.

It was in the repeated visits that I began to recognize and relate to certain paintings and sculptures. If I imagined myself to be a crude but sentient probe being sent into orbit around an unknown planet, then in my loop, my antenna received different and discrete stimuli. I was surprised to find I didn't really care for "funk" art. Even though funk art is "figurative"—featuring recognizable things such as fish and words—I wasn't drawn to it. Not yet anyway. My reaction was the opposite: to hurry past.

But I found myself seeking out the bench in front of Pollock's *Lucifer* and Rothko's *Pink and White over Red*. The scientist in me recognizes my bias here: These are well-known artists, their works the jewels of the collection, and the benches strategically placed. Still, I believe it was more than that: I was also responding to the inherent appeal of these paintings, even though the words to explain why didn't come easily.

On Thursdays I have the great privilege of making afternoon rounds with the three chief residents in internal medicine at Stanford Hospital. They often have a patient in mind for the four of us to see. These sessions are about reading the patient's body as a text, about bettering our skills at mining the body for all it is saying. But we make all sorts of diversions, and one afternoon, in lieu of the bedside, I took them to the Anderson Collection. I made no claim to knowledge or purpose. I wasn't the tour guide—I just walked them through a space that was new to them. In doing so, I thought of a connection to our clinical work: I drew an analogy to the phenomenon of "transference" and "countertransference" in patient care. In psychiatry, for example, patients can develop feelings for the therapist; this transference is often useful for patient and therapist to dissect. Countertransference refers to the feelings the therapist develops for the patient, feelings that range from anger to attraction. Such feelings are normal and important to recognize in oneself, primarily so as not to act on them. Walking among these paintings and observing our responses—both positive and negative—was a means of being self-aware and attentive to a variety of countertransference.

After nearly a dozen visits, alone and with others, even though I wasn't consciously trying to relate the art to the pedagogy of medicine, I began to make connections. My tool is the medical gaze, the desire to look for pathology and connection, and it would seem there was no opportunity for that within a pigmented square of uniform color or a rectangle of haphazard paint splashes. But in me a profound and inward sort of observation was taking form.

Pollock's piece, *Lucifer*, had a manic energy, a seduction—not unlike some hypomanic people I know. (We all know them; they seem more prevalent than they really are, such is their energy.) The force was confined to an elongated rectangle against a white wall. I could imagine the frenzy of an artist standing over the canvas—no easel here—throwing paint at it, using different colors, using anything *but* a brush (turkey basters, syringes). At times I felt I was looking into a mind—*his*, or maybe mine—and seeing the neurofibrillary tangle. It was not the mind depicted in the static histology slides of medical school; it was dynamic and alive, like watching thoughts emerge from a substrate of neurons, or a dream evolving. Yet there was order in the midst of that anarchy. From a distance, the random splashes of color looked mostly black and green, and only when you got close could you see thin streaks of vibrant yellow and blue and red, which were nonetheless necessary for the energy perceived from afar. My response to *Lucifer* was far from constant; it seemed to have a connection with how *my* day had gone.

As my visits accrued, I felt much like someone returning to a city over a long time span. On each visit I noticed that I had changed, and what I observed was changing too.

At first I had studiously avoided reading anything about the art. The rationale was this: In bedside physical exam rounds with my medical students on Wednesdays and chief residents on Thursdays, I ask that if at all possible, the physician or the student who knows the patient, and is bringing us to visit, *not* tell us anything medical about the patient—especially the diagnosis. This isn't so we can be clever and deduce this on our own but rather to ensure that on these rounds (which are not about management, but observation) we are not biased by a label. We can read the body as a sacred text being opened for the first time. Labels such as "cirrhosis" or "endocarditis" can blind us to what else is on display. Similarly, with the paintings, I had wanted to experience them without bias. Now that they were becoming familiar, I read about whatever work caught my fancy.

In 1956 Pollock wrote of his work:

> When I am in my painting, I'm not aware of what I'm doing. It is only after a sort of "get acquainted" period that I see what I have been about. I have no fears about making changes, destroying the image, etc., because the painting has a life of its own. I try to let it come through. *It is only when I lose contact with the painting that the result is a mess.* Otherwise there is pure harmony, an easy give and take, and the painting comes out well.

The italics are mine—that line resonated with me because it paralleled the dystopia that is prevalent in American health care. It's the thing that is dragging down the experience of patients and physicians alike: the sense of *losing contact*. More specifically, it's the sense that the intermediary of the electronic medical record (EMR) and fulfilling every "Lean" mandate has made us lose contact with our work. The result is a mess, with great unhappiness in the ranks.

Rothko's *Pink and White over Red* is a square of a beautiful and vibrant red with a long, horizontal pink rectangular slit at the top, like the slot in the door of a speakeasy as depicted in a noir film— the opening through which the bouncer checks you out. It's the sort of painting that when I was young and ignorant I might have been tempted to dismiss. ("Big deal, I could've done that." The older me might have replied, "Yes, but you would never have thought of it.") But having learned to sit with the painting, to be present, I viewed it differently. It seemed to represent my interior space, what I see on the back of my eyelids when I close my eyes, the image still etched with the glow of the window through which I was gazing. It is soothing. It is the womb. It is emotion. It is preconsciousness.

In the most cursory reading of Rothko, I came across this: "If you are only moved by color relationships, then you miss the point. I'm interested in expressing the big emotions—tragedy, ecstasy, doom." And: "Art is an adventure into an unknown world, which can be explored only by those willing to take the risks."

Forgive me if I felt he was speaking to me personally, rewarding me for being brave enough to drop in from the parking lot and engage with his work. There was also pointed instruction here. If we were to substitute the word "medicine" for "art," his aphorism would read: "Medicine is an adventure into an unknown world, which can be explored only by those willing to take the risks."

Being with patients, being *present* and willing to engage directly in the manner they most want, is a form of risk. The representation of the patient in the EMR (the iPatient, as I call it) is necessary. But being with the iPatient too long is a guaranteed way of *not* being present with the actual patient. It can even begin to feel safer and simpler to be present with one of the many "enchanted objects" around us—computer screens, tablets, and smartphones—than with human beings. Perhaps this is what I most want to teach at the bedside: not the causes of low sodium or the latest sepsis protocol. Or not *just* that (and besides, odds are you can find that online in a flash). I want to teach the art of being present. That, as Rothko says, is an adventure into a risky, unknown world.

I look back and think of patients long gone, particularly patients in the early AIDS era, who were young men for the most part at a time when I, too, was a young man. Was I present? They were full of the ripening of life, full of desire and longing and ambition, at a time when I was full of those things also. I wanted to "do" for them, to fix what ailed them. I wanted to be busy with them in a medical way, even though in those days we had no effective HIV medications and there was nothing we could do to change the course. I would examine them because that was what I knew to do, and that ritual, with its laying on of hands, conveyed an important message to the patient that they would not be abandoned. The absence of any treatment also taught us physicians powerful lessons. I learned from my physician assistant, Della, a warm and caring woman who felt less of the pressure to *do* and instead could just *be*. I remember her cajoling me to make more home visits. Once as we walked in to see a patient who was hours from exiting the world, I said, "What are we going to do here, Della?" She said, "We are going to be with him."

As the German philosopher Martin Heidegger said, sometimes words and speech (and action, I might add) are just a way of forgetting our being or that of the person we are dealing with. I don't think I got it then. I get it now.

Recently, while on rounds with my students, we visited with a patient whose mother was in the room. They were both so gracious, and as ill as he was, he was generous in allowing us to examine him, to focus on aspects of his illness that had little to do with management but were purely to educate the students. Once we were in the hallway, I asked the students if they had noticed anything special about the mother. They had not. And yet the mother had vitiligo, a condition that strips the skin of pigment, a patchy process at first that eventually results in no pigment anywhere for most people with the disease. While it had no bearing on the son's condition, it was a striking observation because the son had darker skin and the mother was almost white. Had we entered as true beginners without homing in on the label "patient," they might have seen it too.

That sense of starting with a blank slate is a feeling I relish. It has become harder to come by. Increasingly, students have a "flipped" patient experience, where a "new" patient is someone they have already met in the computer, having read all their labels *before* seeing them in the flesh. It is as far from the blank canvas as one can get.

My colleague Alexander Nemerov, an art historian and Stanford professor, recently gave the "First Lecture" at the university—an occasion when all thousand-plus Stanford freshmen gather in Memorial Auditorium on their first academic day to hear from a chosen faculty member. In his lecture, Nemerov spoke of Helen Keller, who at 19 months experienced a febrile illness and subsequently lost sight, hearing, and therefore speech. She was in darkness until a remarkable teacher, Anne Sullivan, came into her world.

Nemerov described his visit to the Keller home in Alabama, and to the now-famous water pump on the property, as if visiting a shrine. There, after months of struggling to teach Keller language through signing, Sullivan had held the young girl's hand under the flowing liquid of a hand pump and repeatedly signed out the word "water" in her palm. Suddenly, she broke through. The child understood, as Nemerov says, that the "word and the world could almost magically be the same thing."

I resonated with the image of Keller at the pump. It seems to me that our efforts as teachers are encapsulated in that moment: Our job is to allow the student to "see" in this way, to open up their world.

What is it I want my students to see? I want them to see the signs of disease, the phenotypic manifestations of disease that get buried by the hype around genotype. I want them to see that the outline of a cigarette packet in the shirt pocket of a male patient tells us much more about the patient's risk of sudden death than anything in his genome. So much of diagnosis is to be found in the history and the physical, which in turn guides us to order tests more judiciously. Those visits to the bedside with my students every Wednesday and Thursday—guiding hands to feel spleens and eyes to observe neck veins—are like putting their palms under the water pump, allowing them to feel and connect.

Beyond that there is another kind of seeing that is even more important. Disease is easier to recognize than the individual with the disease, but recognition of the individual whose care is entrusted to us is vital to both parties. There are some simple rules: First, we must go to the bedside, for that is where the patient is. It's a vital and simple step but harder than it looks. It simply isn't possible for the patient to feel recognized and cared for when they feel unattended; the fact that their data is getting a lot of attention in a room full of computer monitors where doctors sit does not satisfy. The gravitational forces of the hospital are always pulling us away from the patient to a screen, and it is not our doing. We are chained to the medical record, and every added keystroke adds another link in the chain. We must be unchained.

Second, when we go to the patient, it follows that we must *listen*, and we must examine with skill. The patient's disease is not located on an image in the computer, nor on a histology slide, nor in numbers of body chemicals—it is located in or on her body. To touch the place that hurts, to examine the body, is to affirm the locus of her illness.

Third, one must revisit and revisit, as few things are completely revealed at the first encounter.

The crises in health care—spiraling costs; inequities of care; the abysmal incentives for primary care; the paucity of geriatric care when our population is aging; physician depression, dissatisfaction, and attrition—offer no easy solutions. There are a few things that are timeless in medicine, unchanged since antiquity, which we can keep front and center as we bring about reform. One is the simple truth that patients want us to be more present. We as physicians want to be more present with the patient as well, because without that contact, our professional life loses much of its meaning.

It is a one-word rallying cry for patients and physicians, the common ground we share, the one thing we should not compromise, the starting place to begin reform, the single word to put on the placard as we rally for the cause.

Presence.

Period.

Rethinking the Traditional Doctor's Visit

A physician and a patient find the missing element for healing in an alternative model of care: shared medical appointments.

Maureen A. Mavrinac

It is a Monday morning in the spring of 2017. The hot, dusty expanse of the Central Valley of California lies below me as the twin-engine plane I'm riding in dips and then swings onto an asphalt runway that separates walls of pistachio trees that are standing so close to one another it looks like they're holding hands.

At the start of each week, I commute from Los Angeles to this remote location, a half hour or more from the nearest ambulance dispatch center and over an hour from the nearest hospital, to work in a start-up clinic that was built by and located within an agricultural company. The area is far from the storied celebrity enclaves of Southern California. During the workweek I stay in company-owned housing in a dusty village with a mostly Latino population. Having attended medical school in Mexico, I am committed to caring for this population.

The clinic, which I worked with from the fall of 2015 until the summer of 2017, is dedicated to reducing the burden of diabetes and reversing the incidence of prediabetes in a largely Latino population of factory and farm workers.

Throughout my career, from my residency in a large inner-city hospital to my current role as a senior primary care physician, I have been frustrated with the one-on-one visit model. I have often felt powerless and hopeless in caring for underserved patients with chronic diseases in the traditional hamster wheel of the 15–20 minutes allotted for individual encounters.

Volume 37, Number 2. February 2018.
Editor's Note: Names have been changed to protect people's privacy.

One day it occurred to me that perhaps the hopelessness I felt was mirrored in the feelings of my patients. Wasn't there a better way to care for patients with chronic disease, a different model that would improve care as well as bring back joy in clinical practice?

"What's missing?" I asked myself.

Failure of the Traditional

After the plane lands, I step gingerly down the stairs and onto the tarmac, hoisting my backpack that is full of groceries for the week. The nearest large supermarket is more than 30 miles away.

Leaving the airport for the clinic, I spray the windshield washer and run the wipers on my small white company car, clearing off the layer of weekend dirt.

"Mariana's here," Julie, one of the medical assistants, announces as I walk into the team room. "She had an appointment Friday, but forgot."

Mariana, a woman in her late 50s, works as a janitor in the agricultural company where the clinic is based. She has never been to school and can't read. She lives alone in a rural hamlet, has no cell phone, and depends on her coworkers to give her a ride to her job each day.

She really doesn't understand diabetes, the disease that now ravages her body. The same disease has affected the lives of close family members. She knows only that it has something to do with *azúcar* (sugar) in the blood, she says. Mariana's idea of self-management for diabetes is "not eating too many foods that taste sweet."

Jen, the clinic's nurse practitioner, and I have struggled for almost a year to care for Mariana and help her care for herself, despite her spotty visits and inaccessibility via phone. We are committed to caring for this underserved population, but we find ourselves more and more overwhelmed with the needs of patients like Mariana who are isolated, have economic challenges, lack formal education, and have ingrained cultural ideas that contribute to poor health literacy.

Culturally sensitive health coaches are assigned to high-risk patients with severely uncontrolled diabetes, including Mariana. But despite best intentions, the one-on-one visits with a coach have not been successful in improving Mariana's glucose control. The goal for most people with diabetes is a hemoglobin A1c level of seven or less. Mariana's consistently runs around 13.

I scroll through Mariana's electronic medical record. A recent screening report shows severe retinal damage, caused by the diabetes. Mariana's health coach, Manny, sighs as he sits down next to me in the team room. He tells me he's reached out to Mariana a number of times, leaving messages with a daughter-in-law without any response. Jen joins us. She has ordered a new insulin pen for Mariana, hoping it will help. None of us are confident in Mariana's ability to manage her medication: There's something else going on here, beyond difficulties of managing medications or getting to doctor appointments. I see it in Mariana's face as I join her in the exam room. She's demoralized.

Rolling the exam stool near the chair where Mariana sits, I study her flat, dull expression. I praise her for coming in and having gone to her eye appointment.

Her eyes fill with tears. "*Doctora*, they told me I could go blind!"

I reach for her hand. I tell her that Manny, Jen, Julie, and I are there to help her and that reducing her blood glucose would help prevent further damage.

Like a good student who wants to please, Mariana tells me that she has been checking her blood sugar at home, and it is running 120 to 180. I find that hard to believe, given Mariana's difficulty with reading and manipulating the glucometer as well as her most recent A1c of 13. That A1c level reflects blood glucose of 326.

I ask Mariana if her son has purchased a cell phone for her yet, as she had previously reported he might. She sniffs, her face red and splotchy, and chokes back tears. She recounts how busy her son is, how her children really don't know how sick she is, and how she doesn't want to burden them.

I offer her a tissue. As she blows her nose and dabs at her eyes, I begin to feel a familiar sinking feeling. I am running out of options for her.

In my days as a clinical preceptor, I witnessed the same dilemma when working with residents. They would plop down next to me, heave a deep sigh, and speak with hopelessness about treating the triad of diagnoses in patients who presented with diabetes, hypertension, and hyperlipidemia. They'd spend a long time discussing diet and medication adherence with their patients, yet they wondered if anything was "sinking in." Invariably, a medical assistant would interrupt and remind the resident that the next patient was outside the exam room, pacing the hall, irritated with the delay.

Thus, the Marianas of the world remain depressed, overwhelmed, and sick. And their clinicians remain powerless, frustrated, and burned out.

Until we don't.

Manny knocks on the exam room door and steps in. He carries with him a brightly colored flyer announcing an upcoming shared medical appointment, a type of appointment where several patients with common health care needs meet together with one or more health care providers. Unlike a traditional one-on-one doctor's visit, shared medical appointments can last one to two hours.

We call our shared medical appointment program Juntos Podemos (which means "together we can"). It's specifically tailored to help address the hopelessness and helplessness of both patients and clinicians in dealing with diabetes. Juntos Podemos usually includes 8 to 15 patients, and it couples brief medical exams, prescription refills, and other medical care with education on topics such as the complications of diabetes. But at the crux of the program is peer interaction and sharing experiences, strength, and hope—akin to a twelve-step program.

I lean forward and look into Mariana's eyes. Manny sits down.

"I want you to come to this," I say to Mariana, pointing to the flyer in Manny's hand. "I know we talked about this group in the past, but now, more than ever, I would love to see you in our next session."

"We can help you get a ride," Manny emphasizes.

We have been down this road before, and Mariana has declined to participate in Juntos Podemos in the past. But today she dabs her eyes and nods. "Yes, I will come."

Together We Can

I have always believed that being a physician is a calling, a vocation. Part of my vocation as a clinician is finding innovative ways to reach patients and help them in their journey toward health. Yet instead of feeling like innovators, many physicians are simply burnt out. Experts consider a loss of agency and control in the processes of health care delivery to be a driving factor.

I feel as if we can reclaim that sense of agency.

In a recent article on the American Academy of Family Physicians website, Victoria Boggiano, a medical student, stated that what attracts her to primary care family medicine is the opportunity to be creative. It is this sense of idealism and passion to innovate that we must preserve and nurture throughout a clinician's professional life.

Shared medical appointments are one creative model for primary care delivery. I became aware of the innovation when I read about the work of Clinica (formerly Clinica Campesina), a federally qualified health clinic in the Denver, Colorado, area. Clinica began to use shared medical appointments more than a decade ago, first with diabetes and then with prenatal care. Cleveland Clinic and Kaiser Permanente also pioneered the model.

It wasn't until 2011, when I began to create shared medical appointments myself while working at an inner-city clinic in Los Angeles, that I understood and finally could articulate what was missing in health care, especially for patients with chronic disease and their clinicians. To me, the shared medical appointment speaks to the soul of our vocation as primary care clinicians in engaging patients, families, and communities.

Our shared medical appointment block consists of six or seven weekly sessions that I run with Manny. Each session covers a specific

topic, such as living with diabetes, managing medications, and dealing with complications of the disease.

Manny is especially energetic on Juntos Podemos days. He preps
the community room, creating a semicircle of tables and chairs to accommodate our patients for the hour-long session. He works with
Julie to collate the patients' latest lab results and gathers up folders
that contain consent forms, handouts, notebooks, and name tags.

As patients arrive, they help each other weigh in and check their
blood pressures with an automatic blood pressure monitor. Julie
checks finger-stick glucose for each of the patients.

Today, two weeks after Mariana agreed to join the first session of
the new appointment block, she appears. I talk about the importance
of helping each other in the journey toward health, and I use the
words "there are unseen people in the room" who will also benefit
from the patient's participation. They get it.

"My grandchildren, my children, my wife—I'm getting healthy for
them and for me," a number of patients say. While Manny encour-
ages participants to share stories, I perform the brief exams, checking their hearts, lungs, and feet.

After the exams, we go around the room discussing A1c levels.

It is a sort of roll call.

"Victor?"

"Seven point zero."

"Ana?"

"Seven point nine."

"Suzy?"

"Five point nine—I'm prediabetic."

"Mariana?"

"I don't know," she says quietly.

Mariana is holding her lab results, but she cannot read. Suzy, a
peer and coworker sitting next to her, leans over to look at Mariana's lab result circled on the sheet.

"OK if I say it?" she asks Mariana. Mariana nods.

"It's thirteen," Suzy replies.

There is a collective gasp. Hearing the astonishment of her peers, Mariana tears up. She tells the group that the eye doctor said she may lose her vision. Manny urges everyone to quietly focus on how "we are all here to help each other."

Mariana is trying to get control of her diabetes, I tell them. We discuss how she struggles with the lack of a phone, an isolated living situation, and long working hours.

At the end of that session, I ask the participants to buddy up during the week to help support each other. Suzy puts her arm around Mariana's shoulders. "I will be Mariana's buddy," she says. "We work in the same area. I will help her."

For the next seven weeks, Mariana and Suzy attend the shared medical appointments together. During that time, Mariana's son finally purchased a cell phone for her as well, at Suzy's urging. After each group session, Jen, Julie, and Manny watch Mariana using the new insulin pen we got for her. They help correct a glaring error: Mariana had been removing the pen before the total dose of insulin was delivered.

At the end of this block of shared medical appointments, it is time to look at A1c values again. When it's Mariana's turn, Suzy reads the result and whispers the number into Mariana's ear.

"Eight point seven," Mariana announces proudly.

The group erupts in applause. They're in a celebratory mood, and for good reason. Many members have seen reduced A1c and weight loss as a result of participating in Juntos Podemos.

Mariana and Suzy sit in the lobby afterward and talk about how much working together has meant to them. They even ask to give a testimonial.

As I hold my phone to record their exchange, Manny, Julie, and Jen look on with wide grins.

Suzy looks at the camera and begins: "Mariana is a good person, a wonderful worker, and I was so happy to help her. You know, it helped me, too. I found myself putting down the extra tortilla when I called to check on Mariana's dinner!"

Then Mariana, fighting back tears, speaks. "I am glad Suzy called me," she says, looking at her friend. "She would call me in the morning and give me a ride to work. We ate lunch together, and at night she would call me and ask what I ate and if I took my medication. I began to have more energy, and really I feel so happy that I have this friend to support and help me. I know I will keep it up because she cares. She has been like a gift."

As I turn off the camera on my phone, it occurs to me that Juntos Podemos has given Mariana, Suzy, Jen, Manny, Julie, and me something that is too often in short supply in primary care.

It has given us hope.

An Urgent Matter

Although the shared medical appointment model has been around for at least a decade, it is not widely implemented—primarily because physicians' schedules and metrics are all built around the one-on-one face-to-face visit. This points to one of the biggest obstacles to starting and sustaining use of the shared medical appointment model: the lack of understanding and support by health system administrators.

In a March 2017 perspective in the *New England Journal of Medicine*, Kamalini Ramdas and Ara Darzi discuss four crucial components that need to be studied to make this innovative model of health care delivery a standard of care. What's needed are rigorous scientific evidence supporting the value of shared appointments, easy ways to pilot and refine shared-appointment models before applying them in particular care settings, regulatory changes or incentives that support the use of such models, and patient and clinician education, they write.

It was not lost on me that their article followed two poignant pieces published in that same March 2017 edition of the *New England Journal of Medicine* about depression and suicide in medical students and physicians. The link between innovation in medicine and finding meaning and joy in practice is clear.

How we deliver primary care is as urgent a matter for clinicians as it is for our patients.

As we learn more about the shared medical appointment model, perhaps we should study an additional component as well: the power of the shared medical appointment in promoting hope both in the patient and in the clinician.

By fostering interpersonal connections and relationships, Juntos Podemos resulted in more effective disease management and better health outcomes for Mariana. It also restored to us, her clinical team, a sense of agency and autonomy, so essential for preventing or reversing burnout.

In the past, my patients' hopelessness mirrored my own.

Now their hope reflects mine.

In the Safety Net

A Tale of Ticking Clocks and Tricky Diagnoses

In a time-crunched clinic, a physician and her resident battle the clock to uncover a potentially fatal diagnosis.

Maria Maldonado

The tempo had been building since our clinic session began. It was a typical Thursday afternoon in February, and the din was rising in the clinic's conference room as our internal medicine residents traded patient stories and plans for dinner, waiting for their turn to present their patients to the attending physicians. I was supervising the internal medicine residents that day, along with one of my colleagues.

Stationed at my computer, I stared at the schedule, unsuccessfully willing it to rearrange itself: Thirty patients on the list, and we were only halfway done. I shook my head. It didn't seem that the visits would be straightforward, either. No one on the schedule appeared to have a routine concern, such as a sore throat or a cold. They were

Volume 32, Number 8. August 2013.

patients with poorly controlled diabetes, requiring medication adjustments; patients with complicated pain syndromes, warranting narcotic medications; or patients with high blood pressure who hadn't taken their medication in months.

The conference room was the inner sanctum of our clinic, a federally qualified health center, where residents-in-training learned the fundamentals of ambulatory care. My colleagues and I who supervise the residents are responsible for the primary care needs of a medically underserved population in Stamford, Connecticut. Rows of shelves containing primary care textbooks and patient information brochures on managing diabetes, hypertension, and high cholesterol in English and Spanish lined the walls of the conference room. Beneath the shelves were corkboards where we pinned telephone lists of community behavioral health centers and community centers, information about accessing phone interpretation, and pamphlets on resources for victims of domestic violence. The doors on either side of the room were kept closed to protect patient confidentiality and to shield us from the glares of angry patients, frustrated by the long waits.

I felt a prickling irritation in my chest as I thought of the clinic's administrative decision to schedule 40-minute appointment slots for new patients and 20-minute slots for follow-up patients. Not enough time, I thought, to decipher the medical needs of our patients, many of whom have limited English proficiency and low health literacy. Not enough time to deal with their lack of work or social supports, exposure to violence in their neighborhoods, impending homelessness, or strategies for managing loneliness and depression with alcohol and drugs. There was never enough time. One could spend hours with these patients before getting to the bottom of their symptoms.

That afternoon, the most essential thing we managed to provide to one particular patient was a bit of extra time. Today I still think of what the consequences could have been if we had not taken that time. We would have missed the opportunity to intervene at a critical moment—and to save our patient's life.

Can I Tell You About a Patient?

One of the residents abruptly brought me out of my reverie. "Can I tell you about a patient?" she asked. The 26-year-old resident was an exceptionally smart, conscientious, and thorough physician-in-training, and I knew that her assessment of her patient would be comprehensive and concise. This time, however, she seemed unusually uncertain. "I think what's going on with this patient is that she's anxious, but something doesn't feel right," she began. "I don't want to blow this off as just depression and anxiety."

She continued to present details about the patient's history and symptoms to me. The patient was a Spanish-speaking 62-year-old woman who was following up at the clinic after a recent emergency department visit, where she had been diagnosed with anxiety and treated with the antianxiety and insomnia drug Ativan. But the medicine wasn't helping at all, the resident explained. For two weeks the woman had had weakness in her right arm. "But I don't find anything unusual on exam," the resident told me, seeming anxious herself. "The patient is worried and is hoping that her symptoms are due to increased stress." Our patient lived alone. She had lived with her daughter until a year ago, when she moved out because her daughter and son-in-law were having marital difficulties. The resident had performed the appropriate neurologic exam, which tests the fitness of the woman's muscle strength and her reflexes, and everything seemed normal.

I knew there were still some additional neurologic tests to be performed to ensure that nothing was physically wrong with our patient, but anxiety seemed to be the leading cause of her symptoms. Many of our immigrant patients experience depression and anxiety that shouldn't be underestimated, I told my resident. The intractable loneliness and sadness that many feel from being separated from family members often translate into chest pain; headache; shortness of breath; and chronic, unremitting pain. Nevertheless, I could tell that the resident wanted me to confirm her findings.

Lately, I also had become more hesitant about attributing symptoms to a psychological cause. One month earlier, after weeks of hoping that my mother's disinterest, weepiness, and lack of concentration were symptoms of depression, we learned that these symptoms were actually warning signs of a malignant brain tumor. She was diagnosed after I finally convinced her to seek medical attention. When my resident came to me that afternoon, I couldn't help but think of my mother.

That day, other residents were waiting to present their patients to me, but I tamped down my sense of urgency so I could be fully present for this patient and my resident. I followed my resident into the exam room, where she introduced me to the woman: petite, with gold-rimmed glasses and blonde hair, which I assumed was dyed. I greeted her in my limited Spanish, while my resident picked up the phone and called for a Spanish interpreter. The interpreter arrived in two minutes. When the wait for an interpreter is long, as it often is, we all smile and nod at each other politely for 10 minutes or more. If the patient speaks Spanish, I ask the very basic questions that I've learned over the years. Given my surname, olive-tan complexion, brown eyes, and dark curly hair, patients assume that I speak Spanish fluently, but I grew up in an English-speaking household. My father, a second-generation Puerto Rican, spoke Spanish, but my mother, the daughter of two Russian immigrants, spoke only English and a bit of Yiddish.

Our patient seemed younger than her 62 years, neatly dressed in trousers and a brightly colored floral blouse. She wasn't overtly nervous. She smiled warmly, but her worry was faintly apparent in the lines of her forehead.

"Can you tell me more about what's going on with you?" I asked the patient, the interpreter echoing my words in Spanish. "You've had this right-arm weakness and difficulty walking, and you think stress is causing the problem? Tell me more about that stress."

The patient's eyes filled with tears. "Well, my daughter is separated from her husband, and I'm worried about her," she answered in Spanish. "I'm not working, and so I can't help her financially."

I waited for the translator.

"How long ago did your daughter get separated?" I asked.

"One year ago," she said.

The timeline didn't make much sense, I thought. A stressful circumstance that began a year ago, and symptoms that started in the past two weeks? As I puzzled, the patient added, "Oh, and one other thing that I forgot to tell the other doctor. I'm not sure this means anything. The other day I was typing, and I couldn't remember where the keys were."

The resident and I exchanged uneasy glances. The history was becoming more ominous. Again I thought of my mother's recent diagnosis. I made a conscious effort to keep my expression neutral, and although I was aware that we were spending more time in the room than I had intended, time had slowed to a stop, at least for me. Out of the corner of my eye, I noticed that my resident kept surreptitiously checking her watch. She was no doubt thinking of the other patients she still needed to see that day, the notes she still needed to write, or her dinner plans that would likely need to be pushed back.

Further Examination

In the exam room, I repeated parts of the neurological exam that my resident had already performed. When I asked her to resist me as I pulled her arm toward me, testing her right-arm strength, she did just fine. But when we asked her to walk down the hallway in the corridor outside the exam room, something my resident had not done, we noticed that she hugged her right arm close to her body, while the left arm swung naturally at her side. The resident and I glanced at each other again, a warning bell ringing in our minds. We escorted the patient back into the exam room, telling her we'd be back shortly, and the resident and I stepped out to discuss the plan.

The next step was to get an imaging study of the patient's brain: either a computed tomography (CT) or magnetic resonance imaging (MRI) scan. A stroke was a possibility, as was a brain tumor. If it was a stroke, we were already too late to provide any treatment that would assuage the acute problem and reverse her right-arm weakness and memory loss. The patient had no medical insurance, so we weighed the costs heavily. A CT scan would be less expensive than an MRI. However, if the scan was unrevealing, then the patient would eventually need the MRI. We decided to refer her for the MRI and to schedule a follow-up visit in a week to discuss the test results.

The resident returned to the exam room to explain the plan to the patient, and the interpreter was brought in again to discuss the next steps. As I began to make my way back to the conference room to meet with my other residents, one of them intercepted me in the corridor to discuss a new patient who had been impatiently waiting for her turn to receive care for a comparatively routine matter. Our patient's 20-minute appointment had lasted over an hour.

Four days after her initial visit, the patient had her MRI. Later that day, my colleague in clinic received an urgent call from the radiologist. Two brain tumors were found, with evidence of brain swelling. In the end, our cautious and deliberate investigation had uncovered a medical emergency. My colleague found an interpreter and quickly called the patient at home, advising her to go immediately to the emergency department, where steroids could be given to alleviate the brain swelling. The patient's brain tumors were caused by metastatic spread of a primary tumor in her lung, we later learned. She underwent brain surgery to have her tumors resected at once, while the tumor in her lung would later be treated with chemotherapy by her oncologist. I didn't see the patient again until six months later, when she returned to our clinic for follow-up. She was feeling "just fine," she said, without any complaints. I was happy and relieved that she was adjusting to her diagnosis and treatment and that she had made it this far. I couldn't help thinking how it could have gone another way.

Our Challenge and Mandate

My colleagues and I often discuss the difficulties of providing patient-centered care to the complex patient population typical of federally qualified health centers such as ours. Many days it feels as if we're hurtling from one patient to the next, hoping that we're delivering the best care possible while effectively teaching our residents. But not every patient's diagnosis and treatment fits neatly in a 20- or 40-minute appointment. Making the right diagnosis in this case required time for translation and investigation to follow the clues that led to our patient's life-saving diagnosis.

The Institute of Medicine says that *high-quality care* is defined in part by a patient-centered focus that includes smooth coordination and timely access. The Accreditation Council for Graduate Medical Education (ACGME) expects residency programs to teach their residents to identify and incorporate patients' preferences into shared decision-making and to seek and fully understand each patient's unique needs, based on culture, ethnicity, sex, and religion.

In safety-net settings, there is often little time to appropriately address the twin challenges of limited English proficiency and low health literacy. These pressures are particularly difficult to balance while also pursuing our educational mission. It is well known that safety-net facilities face unique challenges: Medically underserved patients are more likely than others to have persistent psychiatric problems, drug and alcohol addiction, and unstable economic circumstances that make it difficult to achieve optimal treatment. After years of delaying care for financial reasons or because of their immigration status, many of our patients present with complex chronic illnesses and in advanced stages of disease. Finally, uninsured and underinsured patients often lack access to specialty care. In our clinic, it is fairly typical for our physicians to handle chronic illnesses that in other health care settings are usually managed by specialists. Furthermore, physicians who care for safety-net populations frequently burn out. They may become less empathetic to patients, compromising the quality of care they provide and even exacerbating disparities in their patients' care.

Physicians-in-training often constitute the majority of the workforce in safety-net hospital-based clinics and community health centers. With so little time to devise appropriate solutions to the complex patient scenarios these clinics' residents face, is it any wonder that they later choose careers in specialty disciplines instead of primary care? Most of my own residents have opted for careers in specialties, such as pulmonary/critical care or hospitalist medicine. Perhaps fittingly, the resident who helped me discover this patient's tumors is now applying for a fellowship in hematology and oncology.

The Affordable Care Act attempts to address the looming shortage of primary care physicians willing to work with underserved communities by introducing the Teaching Health Center Graduate Medical Education Program. Implemented in 2011, the program is designed to increase the number of primary care residents training in community-based settings across the United States. Federal graduate medical education funds are funneled to the community health centers participating in the program instead of to hospitals where residency programs are historically seated. The teaching health centers are held accountable for outcomes, such as the number of residents who complete training and continue to deliver primary care to underserved areas. These teaching health centers also typically provide training in cultural competency and community medicine and evaluate residents' ability to deliver competent care to diverse populations.

But establishing a teaching health center is a lengthy process, requiring approval and accreditation by the ACGME. To date, few of these centers have been established, and the Affordable Care Act's funding for them is guaranteed only through 2015.

Of course, funding is not the only force shaping how patients are treated by safety-net providers. The Safety Net Medical Home Initiative, sponsored by the Commonwealth Fund, is committed to transforming 65 community health centers into patient-centered medical homes, emphasizing engaged leadership, quality improvement strategies, continuity of care, evidence-based care, enhanced access, and care coordination. This initiative underscores the need to reward providers for value over volume; to bring the patient-centered medical home model to safety-net settings, payers will need to find a way to appropriately reimburse practices that care for the medically underserved. As one potential model, Minnesota launched a payment program in 2008 that took into account patient complexity, with factors such as limited English proficiency and serious or persistent mental illness triggering additional payment for such patients.

A New Commitment

In the meantime, I think about the messages we are sending to residents about who is entitled to patient-centered care and who is not—not in what we say or teach them, but in the reality they witness and experience. To recruit a new generation of physicians willing to tackle the challenges of the safety net, medical students and residents must be shown that even the most complex patient population must be cared for with compassion, skill, understanding, and, of course, time. Schedules should be devised with regard for the patient's language, complexity of care, and health literacy—instead of imposing arbitrary time limits across the board.

At a time when budgets are stretched thin, most people on the front lines caring for patients find themselves examining how their resources are being used and looking for ways to use them more productively and efficiently. Any discussion of health care resource allocation must begin with the goals we value most as a society. Do we fundamentally believe that everyone has a right to high-value patient-centered care? If so, we must accept that a unique set of barriers separates each patient from the care he or she needs and then build meaningful tools to overcome those barriers.

Medical students and residents form the backbone of the safety-net workforce, and they get their cues from us—medical educators. Based on our example, they develop lifelong attitudes and approaches to their patients. If we want to pass the values of patient-centered care on to our students, we must practice them ourselves. We need resources to do this, and one of the most valuable resources of all is time.

The Personal Toll of Practicing Medicine

A physician and lifelong patient reflects on her truncated career and why the health of experienced doctors needs protection.

Elaine Schattner

If you met me in the mid-1990s, you would have encountered a hard-working, energetic young physician. I was in my 30s; my sons were in elementary school. Most mornings, I left our Manhattan apartment by 7:00 a.m. We lived near the hospitals where my responsibilities included clinical care, research, and teaching. I specialized in blood diseases and cancer, held a tenure-track position, and ran a small laboratory. On good days, I returned home by 7:00 p.m. for dinner with my family. After supper, I stayed up late working and reading.

Those years were filled with long days, interrupted nights, and challenging weekends on call. Sure, I was tired, but I didn't mind. I was happy and excited in my work and took pride in being a physician. My husband was supportive, and my sons didn't seem to mind my demanding career. Quite the opposite: I overheard their occasional boasts that their mom was a doctor and researcher. Several times, when we traveled as a family and someone called for a doctor on an airplane or in an airport, they'd yell: "Mom! You should go help." I always did.

Being a doctor was essential to my identity. It's a hard thing to give up. My father was a physician, and I'd always admired his work and enthusiasm for science. When I became a patient at age six with a scoliotic S-shaped spine, I learned how essential a caring doctor can be. I wore a back brace for four years, but it didn't work. In the end, I needed surgery and a steel rod fused along my spine if I wished to stand properly, walk, or bear children. I stayed five weeks in a hospital for spine-pulling traction and a long operation complicated by a blood clot, followed by 10 months in a body cast, all before my fifteenth birthday. Those experiences affected my career and motivation to help others.

After college, I spent a year working in a lab at Rockefeller University, and at age 23 I entered medical school, also in New York City. I scrubbed in at surgery, helped deliver babies, cared for patients dying from AIDS, and more. During summers, I performed basic research in a cell biology lab at the medical school. I then completed a three-year residency in internal medicine. Next came a three-year fellowship in hematology and oncology. When I completed my training and became faculty at age 33, I was a highly educated woman.

To say that I loved my work is an understatement. I don't think I could have imagined then that I'd be closing a small practice in December 2006, just 13 years after finishing my training. I still miss my work in the clinic, and my lab. The day I saw my last patient was one of the hardest of my life.

When you hear about physicians, particularly in oncology, suffering burnout and depression, practitioners' emotional health gets most of the attention. Those are real problems, and they affected me. I became depressed. But that happened largely after the physical demands of my job took their creeping toll. Being a doctor takes stamina, and I was lacking in that after developing several serious health problems.

A big factor in my decision to stop practicing—and why I share this story, so that it might be addressed—was the intense, physically demanding, and needlessly competitive environment of academic medicine, as well as the pressures of private practice, which I experienced briefly at the end of my clinical career. Neither way of practicing medicine was compatible with my health. Nor is it conducive to anyone's. My intention is not to point fingers toward any individual or institution but to draw attention to the greater issue of physicians' health. It's a delicate subject, fraught with privacy and safety concerns.

Physical Demands, Long Hours

When I began my fellowship in hematology and medical oncology, I was several months pregnant. The pregnancy would be no problem, my division chief assured me. And it wasn't. I recall that July in 1990, walking up steps in the hospital with my team: the attending physician, fellows, a few residents, and a medical student or two. The supervising physician was a workplace wellness pioneer; he always took the stairs. "How's the pregnant member of the team doing?" he called out, looking down from two flights above. He seemed genuinely concerned.

"I'm fine," I answered, and continued walking.

But the episode was a flag, I should have realized sooner, for how strenuous working in a large medical center can be. By then it had been 15 years since my scoliosis surgery, and I didn't think about my health. I didn't want to disappoint the physician and mentor I admired. I didn't want to appear weak, to him or my peers.

Late that year I had my baby and took seven weeks of maternity leave. In 1990 that seemed ample. After the birth of my second child two years later, I took three months off from a research rotation. My peers in the training program—friends, really—covered my patients while I was out. They were gracious about it. Some gave gifts.

During both pregnancies, I managed a full caseload and performed bone marrow biopsies, spinal taps, chemotherapy administration, and other procedures. Among the fellows, we rotated who would be on call for nights, weekends, and holidays. A sense of fairness prevailed. Whatever weekends and holidays I missed, before and after giving birth, I would make up in other seasons.

We took turns fielding requests from other doctors to see patients with blood or cancer problems. Some were quite sick and needed evaluation at odd hours. A postoperative patient in the recovery room, hemorrhaging from a major artery, might get a hematology consult at 2:00 a.m. Or a young woman with undiagnosed cancer and excruciating back pain who was losing sensation in her toes because a tumor was causing compression of her spinal cord might need an oncology evaluation at 8:00 p.m. on a Saturday. After consultation, many of the patients came to see us in the clinic and to know us as their physicians. We fellows shared a sense of responsibility for their care.

When I joined the faculty of my academic institution in 1993, my time in the outpatient clinic was nominally limited to a half-day each week, although my responsibilities spilled into evenings with phone calls and daily visits to my hospitalized patients. When I wasn't with patients, most of the time I was working in a lab. My research focused on immune cells called lymphocytes and what can go wrong with those cells in leukemia. In 1996 I received an independent grant from the National Institutes of Health (NIH). That boded well for my career. Meanwhile, I taught students about physical diagnosis, medical ethics, and hematology and gave lectures on lymphoma and immune cell signaling.

For a couple of months each year, I was "on service," which meant I was responsible for hospitalized patients with cancer or blood problems. I'd meet with the team for morning rounds starting around 7:30 a.m., we'd examine all the patients, and then I'd head to the lab, to the outpatient clinic, or to a conference room for teaching. I was required to participate in other activities, including case presentations, grand rounds, and a journal club in which we discussed new science publications. It was a lot of work, but I was constantly learning and enjoyed it!

Weekends on call could be brutal. My pager or cell phone rang nonstop. I remember middle-of-the-night phone calls: from a man whose wife, a patient with breast cancer and brain metastases, was seizing; from medical residents in the intensive care unit who asked me to come in to speak with the elderly European parents of a man who died that night from lymphoma; from an obstetrician seeking guidance for a pregnant woman who lacked platelets and was in labor. The decisions were fast-paced, life-and-death kind of stuff. I put off whatever could wait until Monday morning when my colleagues returned, but many problems could not wait.

Difficult Years

My work was going well until around 1998. I had only one grant from the NIH to support my lab and needed another, but we were having trouble getting our data published in top journals. Around then, I noticed in a family video that I looked bent over, almost like an old woman. It scared me. I was only 38 years old. I began experiencing some back pain, enough that I began swimming laps twice each week to strengthen my back muscles and lessen the discomfort.

In 2001 I lost the NIH grant. To support my lab and salary, I needed to bring in more clinical revenue, so I was assigned to more clinics and additional time on hospital wards. I began seeing a psychiatrist for depression. For most of another year, I tried to keep the lab going, performing experiments requested by reviewers of my grant proposals, and rewriting and resubmitting those. But it was an exercise in frustration; I closed the lab in the summer of 2002.

I was devastated, and I put my heart into clinical work. Seeing patients made me feel better; it boosted my sense of self-worth and took my mind off the searing pain in my lower spine. To relieve my discomfort, I popped maximum doses of Motrin, Tylenol, and Vioxx. But the pain was getting worse and worse. I had a computed tomography (CT) myelogram, a headache-inducing procedure during which neuroradiologists injected dye into my spinal canal to image the surrounding membranes and bones. I didn't tell my colleagues. I was due to give a presentation the next morning, and I did.

The myelogram showed that the vertebrae below the old rod were crumbling. There was almost no cartilage between two pairs of lower vertebrae. I'd need surgery to stabilize the lower spine and prevent further deterioration.

The operation would be dangerous. The orthopedics team would open me up from the front, entering the lower abdomen to insert

titanium cages—like metal cushions—where intervertebral cartilage had been. Then they'd flip me over, open my back, and apply a
steel cutter to sever the old rod that had been fused to my spine
since 1974. I was fully aware of possible complications, as I'd con-
sulted on similar cases at the orthopedics hospital. I feared becoming paralyzed, dying at age 42, or being stuck on a machine (in that
order). I reviewed my end-of-life preferences with my husband and
physicians.

In the midst of pre-op evaluation for that surgery, my internist
noted my age and that I hadn't had a screening mammogram. My
breasts were a bit lumpy and hard to examine because of fibrocystic
changes that are usually benign. What was running through my mind,
then, was that I had no time for breast cancer. I was worried about
my job, and my back. But I generally tried to follow my doctor's advice, so I scheduled the procedure. The image was abnormal, and the
radiologist immediately ordered a sonogram, which revealed a concerning lesion in my left breast. Days later, the radiologist took five
core needle samples. Later that morning, I headed into work with
bandages under my bra, beneath a dark-colored blouse.

It turned out I had a 1.5 centimeter stage I invasive tumor. That
didn't faze me much. As an oncologist, I knew that breast cancer is
usually treatable if caught early. Magnetic resonance imaging also
showed a concerning spot in the right breast. Because of the scoliosis, I wanted to drop weight off my chest and be as symmetric as
possible, so I chose bilateral mastectomy. Given the upcoming spine
surgery, my doctors advised the simplest means of reconstruction,
with tissue expanders that could be exchanged for implants later.

I wore a wig and worked through the four cycles of chemotherapy, which lasted three months. We scheduled treatments on Fri-
days so I could recover on weekends after each infusion. My division chief was supportive, as were most of my colleagues. The
division chief switched the schedule so I'd be away from the hospital floors out of concern that my immune system was compromised
by the chemotherapy. I was assigned more administrative tasks, such

as sitting on a quality-of-care committee. Looking back on those months, I don't think I got much done.

One morning that December, in 2002, I slipped backward on ice on the sidewalk while walking to the pool for a swim. I threw my right arm behind me to protect my back as I fell, and I broke it. From that point forward, I had difficulty writing and typing with my dominant arm.

A radiologist noted from my X-rays that my bones were thin and I probably had osteoporosis. I was becoming numb.

"I can't have another diagnosis," I told friends.

But a bone scan and blood work confirmed osteoporosis. My doctors advised reevaluation and possible treatment later, after the chemotherapy and spine surgery.

The spine operation took place in March 2003. The orthopedists placed two titanium cages in vertebral spaces, put two additional rods and seven bolts along my spine, and inserted a stabilizing screw into my right pelvic bone. I was hospitalized for two weeks and sent home on a prophylactic blood thinner and oral morphine. I wore a back brace and needed a walker. I was assigned a visiting nurse, an aide, and in-home physical therapy. I could not stand up, use the bathroom, or brush my teeth without assistance. Through all of this, my husband, sons, sisters, parents, and friends helped me.

After surgery, I took five months off from work. At home, I watched movies, read books, and studied to recertify in hematology and medical oncology. One thing I regret is that I did not attend any meetings at the medical center with my walker or cane. I was too proud; I didn't want anyone's pity. My hair was slow to return, and I was still wearing the wig. But maybe if my colleagues had seen me then, they would have better understood what I'd gone through and later treated me with greater empathy. Perhaps a supervisor would not have said flippantly, as he did the next year, "I heard you had some kind of back surgery."

The usual time off recommended after the kind of spine operation that I had—without breast cancer—was 6 to 12 months. A supervisor persuaded me to return after five. The charm was that he made me feel needed: two doctors had left the group, and they were short on doctors qualified in hematology. I wanted to be a team player. I hesitated but agreed. A few months later, he took a position elsewhere.

Ending My Practice

When I returned to work, it was a disaster. I had no grant to support my salary and was soon assigned to be on service at the hospital for half of most months. I was often responsible for more than 30 hospitalized patients at any given time, and on weekends that number could exceed 50. Almost every evening, I came home late. I missed dinners. I had no time to finish the reconstruction of my breasts. The chemotherapy had induced early menopause. I was physically and emotionally exhausted.

I asked for a lighter workload. A supervisor suggested I was spending too much time speaking with the hospitalized patients when seeing them faster would make my life easier. He might have been right. After my recent cancer treatment, I was more inclined than ever to answer patients' questions and to treat them with care. Meanwhile, my coworkers were becoming more protective of their time. If I needed a few hours for a medical appointment or procedure, I'd have to ask a colleague to cover for me. Two years after my cancer diagnosis, they were less likely to oblige. Understandably, they wanted to get home to their families or friends too.

Yet my clinical reputation was growing. I had valuable knowledge of rare blood disorders and was receiving more and more referrals of challenging cases. In 2005 I switched to private practice and tried to limit my hours. Toward the end of my practice, patients came from other states and even Canada to see me. But I couldn't manage my work and tend to my own medical needs. I continued to delay fixes to my breast reconstruction. I gained weight. I missed physical therapy and arrived late to sessions with my psychiatrist.

When I finally stopped practicing medicine, I was board-certified in hematology and medical oncology. Yet I felt like a failure and a burden to my colleagues. I had many patients, and one of the hardest things about that experience was not being able to tell them why I closed my practice, because I was so depressed. I felt that I had failed them. I contemplated suicide.

In retrospect, it's clear that the demands placed on me were too great for anyone. No physician, at any age, should be expected to work those kinds of hours. True, I pushed myself too hard and made some bad decisions. I also had some very bad luck. But there was little slack in the system among the group of blood and cancer specialists with whom I worked. That remains a problem for clinicians today. A culture of not complaining—of not "whining" about your hours and schedule, no matter how unreasonable or unsafe those might be—prevails and can press doctors to work beyond what's healthy.

Protecting Our Time

In 2003 the Accreditation Council for Graduate Medical Education (ACGME) implemented work-hour limits for early-career physicians, while some states began restrictions earlier. Most residents and fellows are permitted no more than 24 hours of continuous duty. Residency and fellowship programs must follow these rules to maintain ACGME certification and funding.

Yet few if any rules limit the work hours of experienced doctors. To the best of my knowledge, there's no constraint on how many consecutive hours a neurosurgeon or a consulting hematologist might be on call. As things stand, many senior physicians lack support, backup, or rest.

In 2009 the *American Journal of Medicine* published one of the few academic reports on the hours of practicing physicians. That small study found that some physicians regularly work more than 80 hours per week and more than 30 consecutive hours without rest—exceeding the limits imposed on residents and fellows.

Some organizations that might promote physicians' health, such as state medical societies, sponsor programs for doctors who are (or are suspected to be) impaired because of mental illness, drug, or alcohol addiction. For example, the Medical Society of the State of New York runs a Committee for Physician Health to protect practitioners with substance use and other psychiatric disorders, but the committee does not focus on maintaining the wellness of aging physicians or protecting doctors' time.

Meanwhile, hospitals, employers, and some state licensing boards have upped their requirements for doctors' continuing medical education and board certification. These crucial activities require physicians' time and focus. Practitioners need dedicated hours—and their employers' support—for learning.

Supporting Physicians' Well-Being

I'm not sure if any law or workload regulations would have saved my clinical career. But I do think some changes would benefit others.

A slower expected pace of practicing medicine could support the health of doctors and of their patients. The Aliki Initiative at Johns Hopkins Bayview Medical Center, designed to train resident doctors in a "thoughtful" approach to care, provides an example from which other employers might draw. In that program, some medical residents were assigned half the usual numbers of patients. Preliminary findings indicate that outcomes, such as hospital readmissions after heart failure, may be improved and costs of care may be lowered. Residents in the program report learning more, and patients report improved experiences.

A simple step would be to provide all doctors with adequate clerical support. For years, as faculty, I shared a secretary with other physicians at the medical center. Having my own assistant would have helped me tremendously and might have benefited my patients too. Hiring more expert staff, such as nurse practitioners and physician assistants, also can help patients and doctors, and improve care. But those staff might not be prepared to take on extreme medical problems. Also, I'm wary that excessive reliance on staff tends to diminish relationships between doctors and patients. By spending less time with each patient, a doctor will come to know them less well.

That dissociation diminishes trust (in both directions) and breeds indifference—the opposite of what's needed in medical care.

In some areas of medicine, limiting hours may be irrelevant. Hospitalists and emergency department doctors, for instance, typically work in finite shifts. In dermatology, emergencies occur very rarely. Telemedicine could help (and is already) in some fields, such as cardiology, by permitting doctors in other locations to take on some of the workload. But telemedicine can't supply immediate hands-on care, such as surgery for a ruptured heart valve.

To be sure, an occasional tough weekend on call or consult at 3:00 a.m. will always be necessary. I'm not suggesting that doctors avoid working 10-hour days, 50-hour weeks, and some weekends and holidays. That's the arrangement most of us expected when we applied to medical school. But years of working 60- and 70-hour weeks and covering practices on most weeknights can sap a person's energy and negatively affect well-being.

Physicians at any age would benefit from standard workplace measures to protect their positions should their health decline or they need to take leave. Where there's a lack of support for doctors in those circumstances, the issue can and should be addressed by anti-discrimination and disability regulations. But such rules can't create a more compassionate work environment in and of themselves.

Looking Forward

I'm feeling much better now, overall. I'm happy again. Yet my physical health remains tenuous. Most recently, doctors found a narrowing in my large intestine, and this past August, a colorectal specialist removed a foot-length segment. Fortunately, it turned out benign. I celebrated those results with my husband and now-grown sons. I am healing well and swimming again. I expect to be around to write and teach for some time ahead. And I will continue to rely on the knowledge and well-being of my physicians, whose health matters.

2

Medical Innovation and Research

Cancer, Our Genes, and the Anxiety of Risk-Based Medicine

Advanced medical technologies make it easier to identify people at risk for cancer, but there are risks involved in oversurveillance too.

Siddhartha Mukherjee

In the summer of 2005 I met a woman, Laura M., whose life had been overturned by cancer. But she was disease free: It was the anxiety of cancer in the future that haunted her.

Laura had been diagnosed with a primary tumor in her breast that was small and localized. She had had surgery, radiation, and chemotherapy—a standard treatment protocol—and had then come to see me, an oncologist, to help manage her future care. I suggested doing nothing. Everything about her case suggested a good prognosis: We all agreed that she had likely been cured. But in the wake of her treatment, she became obsessed by the possibility of a relapse. She scoured her family history and discovered a distant aunt who had died of breast cancer at age 70. Her own mother had died at a young age from a car accident, but Laura became convinced that had her mother lived, she would have been diagnosed with breast cancer.

Laura's visits to the clinic were punctuated by her sense of doom. She often came in with sheaves of papers that she had printed from the internet about "occult metastasis," which had been found in patients who, like her, were thought to be at low risk. She repeatedly asked me to confirm that she "had been given the most aggressive chemo regimen that could be given." (She had, in fact, been treated with the appropriate regimen recommended for her case.) We checked her for genetic susceptibilities, such as inherited mutations in the *BRCA1* and *BRCA2* genes that increase cancer risk, but found none.

Volume 37, Number 5. May 2018.
Editor's Note: The patient's name and certain identifying details were changed by the author to protect the patient's privacy.

Nonetheless, she asked if she and her daughter could undergo "the most intensive form of cancer surveillance" to detect early cancers in her body.

Laura's story highlights a new anxiety about illness that is permeating our culture. It is the anxiety of being under constant diagnostic surveillance, of inhabiting a state of vigilant watchfulness for illnesses before they can take root in one's body. It is the state, as one patient described it, of "feeling under siege from the future." Emblematic of this anxiety is the concept of a "previvor"—a strange new term invented to describe a person who is a survivor of an illness that she is predisposed to but has yet to have. For Laura, these states were contiguous: her survivorship from one breast cancer had turned overnight, it seemed, into "previvorship" for another breast cancer.

As I write this, two kinds of technologies are radically altering the landscape of cancer risk and screening. The first involves what we might call "genetic surveillance"—an attempt to quantify an individual's inherited predisposition for cancer (that is, you should be surveyed for the disease because of the higher risk conferred by your genes). The second, in contrast, involves "chemical surveillance"—an attempt to detect chemical markers of incipient cancers in blood (that is, you should be surveyed because there's a sign of early cancer circulating in your blood). The two technologies converge to increase the supply of men and women who are forced to enter the domain of surveillance and screening. Both, in short, encourage men and women without current cancer, but with the prospect of future cancer, to become citizens or permanent residents of what Susan Sontag once described as "the kingdom of the ill."

Genetic Screening and Cancer Risk

For decades, perhaps centuries, we've known of families where some form of cancer (usually the same type: breast or pancreatic) is manifest in multiple individuals across multiple generations. Not every family member is affected, but the risk of cancer in such a family clearly lies beyond the average risk of cancer in the population.

Until recently, our capacity to identify the culprit genes in such families—or, more actionably, to identify the members of the family who carried the heightened risk—was limited to inherited single-gene mutations. These included mutations in genes such as *BRCA1*, *BRCA2*, and *MLH1* that, if inherited from parents, increase the likelihood of breast, colon, and other cancers by severalfold over normal individuals. But many human traits, including cancer risk, might not track with single-gene mutations. Take human height as an example. Height is highly heritable—we know that tall parents tend to produce tall children, and shorter parents bear shorter children—yet early attempts to pin down the variation in human height to single-gene variations or mutations revealed only a smattering of candidate genes. (For this essay, I use the terms "variation" and "mutation" interchangeably, although there are subtle differences.) Geneticists described this conundrum, famously, as the "missing heritability" of height: we could infer from the pattern of inheritance that height-determining genes must exist in the human genome, but their precise identity and number remained unknown.

By similar logic, the inherited risk of cancer might be carried by mutations or variations not in one but in multiple genes, each of which acts together to increase an individual's risk of the disease. In the 1990s, some breast cancer patients began to refer to the next as-yet-unidentified conglomerate of genes for breast cancer as "*BRCA3*." That name carried both a sardonic and a hopeful edge. Unlike patients with definite *BRCA1* and *BRCA2* mutations, patients with potential *BRCA3* mutations remained suspended in an anxious limbo. We could not diagnose a woman with this genetic syndrome yet because we had no idea what these genes might be (a few additional single-gene mutations that increased breast cancer risk were identified in the 2000s, but most patients with breast cancer continued to lack a single-gene explanation). A *BRCA3* patient's experience of her terrifying family history and dread of future disease were just as acute as those of a patient with known cancer-risk mutations, but the genes that precipitated the former patient's fate were hidden from our view. As doctors, we'd acknowledge the risk that these patients carried—with their family histories scarred by breast cancer—but we were unable to offer a more tangible description of their susceptibility to the disease.

This state of suspension for polygenic (or multigene) diseases is finally being relieved: the combinations of gene mutations responsible for such genetically complex diseases are now being identified by powerful computational technologies. Computational algorithms (some involving deep learning or machine learning), in particular, have been unleashed on human genomes. By scanning millions of fully sequenced genomes, these algorithms dissect how variations in thousands of genes, each exerting a small effect, might ultimately add up to the heightened risk of an illness—a problem of such mind-boggling complexity that previous computational technologies had failed to capture it. One algorithm has learned to predict human height as the consequence of variations in a thousand-odd genes. (Take a moment to digest this startling fact: such an algorithm might soon predict your actual height, or the future height of your unborn child, based on your genetic sequence alone.) Another program is learning to predict the risk of cardiovascular disease—again, likely the consequence of hundreds of gene mutations or variations. With such advances, it is likely that an algorithm might identify those of us at highest genetic risk for future cancers. (Of course, for many cancers, even ones that run in families, there's still a powerful influence of chance and the environment. A woman with a *BRCA1* mutation might increase her risk for breast cancer through certain exposures, by virtue of inheriting other "modifier" genes or by chance alone. These additional variables are not yet part of the computational landscape but could become incorporated into algorithms in the future.) This technology, then, could serve as a portal of entry into the world of cancer for potentially millions of men and women who seek to be annotated for future cancer risk and potentially surveyed for cancer.

Advancements in Cancer Detection

While computers seek out patients who have an inherited susceptibility to cancer, other machines are seeking to identify chemicals that
might currently be in our blood or other organs that signal cancer
risk. Termed "liquid biopsy" or "liquid surveillance," these methods
attempt to discover minuscule amounts of the products shed or spilled
by cancer cells—DNA, proteins, and other substances—into the
blood or other circulating tissues. Once such trace signs of an incipient cancer are found, the logic runs, cancer will be detected in its
earliest stages and can be attacked with more effective therapies. We
will scour the body to find ovarian, lung, and prostate cancers, for
instance, before these become clinically manifest, thereby enabling
better treatments.

These liquid biopsies run the risk of overdiagnosing patients, however. What if someone is found to carry a liquid marker for ovarian
cancer, say, but that ovarian cancer never takes root in her body?
Cancer cells, we now know, can exist in a body, or a site within the
body, without becoming manifest as clinical disease or a detectable
metastasis. (Most likely, this is because the "soil" of a particular organ does not allow the "seed" of a cancer to sprout.) Or what if some
of the markers turn out to overlap with benign diseases (as was the
case with earlier liquid surveillance markers, such as the prostate-
specific antigen test for prostate cancer), thereby increasing the risk
of false positive results?

Nonetheless, enthusiasm for the liquid surveillance of cancer seems
to grow exponentially each day (one private company that hopes to
advance this technology goes by the name Grail, emblematic of the
near-religious fervor with which some advocates describe the power
of liquid biopsies). Many patients in my cancer clinic now come to
their appointments armed with brochures about liquid biopsies, won-
dering whether their tumors might have been detected earlier had
such biopsies been performed. These technologies represent a second
portal of entry into the world of cancer. By identifying men and

women who might be bearing the first markers of cancer, these methods increase the pool of those who must be surveyed and further screened for the illness.

The Total Institution of Cancer

My aim is to neither exaggerate nor minimize the transformative potential of these technologies, although it's worthwhile emphasizing this at the outset. The capacity to identify humans with an increased genetic risk for cancer, coupled with the possibility of detecting cancer at its earliest stages using a liquid biopsy, might radically change how we prevent, detect, and treat cancer. But my concern is the effect that such surveillance might have on our bodies and societies. In the 1950s the sociologist Erving Goffman wrote a remarkable article about the concept of a "total institution," an idea that he expanded in subsequent work. "A total institution," Goffman wrote in his 1961 book *Asylums*, is one "where a great number of similarly situated people, cut off from the wider community for a considerable time, together lead an enclosed, formally administered round of life." Total institutions, such as mental hospitals, prisons, and even boarding schools, have rituals of entry and exit. They inculcate belonging. They invent their own vocabulary and codes of behavior; they have an internal logic, impenetrable to others. They encourage surveillance and create anxiety. Members are united by a common sense of purpose, by the feeling of being chosen or marked. Those who are expelled may feel a sense of betrayal, while those who remain can be consumed by the guilt of survivorship.

Cancer, too, runs the risk of becoming a "total institution." A patient, once diagnosed, may be whisked away into a cancer ward, dressed in a patient's smock—"a tragicomically cruel costume, no less blighting than a prisoner's jumpsuit," as I wrote in *The Emperor of All Maladies*—and stripped of his identity. When I once asked a woman with a rare sarcoma about her life outside the hospital, she observed, "I am in the hospital even when I am outside the hospital."

In this new era of cancer treatment, I wonder if we are unwittingly, but insidiously, intensifying the totality of the "cancer institution" for patients. For people like Laura M., cancer has certainly become a total institution—or a "cancer world," as some patients call it. They are in either treatment, remission, surveillance, maintenance, or re-surveillance. Mavens of early detection are also working on deep-learning algorithms that will pick up cancerous lesions on patients' imaging results and classify them as malignant, using criteria that seem to defy even the most acute human eye. In an April 2017 article in the *New Yorker*, I wrote about one of the pioneers of this idea, the German computer scientist Sebastian Thrun. Thrun imagines a world in which even the daily instruments of our normal lives are morphed into weapons of diagnostic surveillance—a bathtub that scans your body to detect abnormal masses that might require investigation; a mirror that could check your body for precancerous moles; a computer program that (with your consent) would scour your Instagram or Facebook page while you slept at night, evaluating changes in your photographs that might signal signs of cancer.

Then there's the question of treatment and cost. If an additional tumor—clinically undetectable, but discovered by these novel methods—were detected in Laura M.'s case and the primary lesion removed, what criteria would we use to determine whether we should use some form of adjuvant (or extra) medicine, such as cell-killing chemotherapy or targeted therapy, after the initial surgical removal, as is often done for most cancers? The costs of such surveillance and treatment—an astronomical amount if every human had to be genetically annotated, subjected to surveillance, and treated if a tumor was found—would overwhelm current projections of medical costs (although in the most optimistic scenario, the benefits would also be amplified in lives saved via early diagnosis). Thorny issues of overdiagnosis and overtreatment would have to be addressed. We would have to devise careful guidelines about when *not* to act and whom *not* to treat.

For Laura M., the answer to each of these questions carries immense consequences. She has entered a strange new world, one of

constant diagnostic surveillance; of dealing with the anxiety of relapse and maintenance; of that peculiar desolation of the shuttle from
clinical trial to clinical trial, and from hospital to hospital, as she tries
to keep one step ahead in this chess game against cancer; and of
watching doctors pit their will, wit, and imagination against a for-
midable enemy that keeps changing its shape. This world has created
its own internal vocabulary. A "haircut party" is a celebration thrown
in honor of a person about to enter the cancer world (as a sign of
solidarity, even if the patient is spared hair-loss inducing chemo). "No
Exit chemo," as a patient of mine put it, describes the fact that a
unique personalized chemo regimen for a patient produces unique
toxicities, a phrase borrowed from the Jean-Paul Sartre novel in
which every human being is assigned his or her own personal hell.

"A world in which cancer is normalized as a manageable chronic
condition would be a wonderful thing," the medical historian Steven
Shapin wrote in a 2010 review of *The Emperor of All Maladies*. "But
a risk-factor world in which we all think of ourselves as precancerous would not," he continued. "It might decrease the incidence of
some forms of malignancy while hugely increasing the numbers of
healthy people under medical treatment. It would be a strange victory in which the price to be paid for checking the spread of cancer
through the body is its uncontrolled spread through the culture."

To date, Laura M. has not suffered from a relapse of breast cancer. Nor, fortunately, has she had a new cancer anywhere in her body.
But the "strange victory" over her body has not spared her mind. She
remains haunted by the future prospect of illness. When Susan Sontag wrote of a passport between the kingdom of the well and the
kingdom of the ill, she imagined a bidirectional passage: men and
women might pass into illness, but some would return to wellness.
In inventing cancer's new surveillance culture, I fear that we have
closed the borders of the kingdoms. I fear that we now possess just
one-way passports into the realm of illness.

Beating a Cancer Death Sentence

A melanoma survivor describes his arduous—and costly—path to successful treatment and hope.

Jonathan Friedlaender

Several months ago, my wife, Françoise, and I attended something novel for melanoma patients: a survivors' dinner. People said they wanted to make it an annual gathering. Planning anything that far in advance had been pointless for me. Two years ago, I was about to accept hospice care.

When I was first diagnosed in 1996, early surgery was the only reliably successful treatment. Anything more advanced was essentially a death sentence. Over the past five years, a series of revolutionary drugs have given me and many other people a surprisingly hopeful prospect. Nevertheless, the drugs' development process has often been excruciating for clinical trial participants, and their remarkably high costs limit their value.

Diagnosis and Early Treatment

I have the most common form of melanoma, which occurs in fair-complexioned people who had blistering sunburns in their youth. I also spent a year in my 20s in the South Pacific, doing biological-anthropological fieldwork, which meant more episodes of particularly intense sun exposure.

My first melanoma lesion revealed itself three decades later—in 1996, when I was 56—as a small irregular raised blue-gray lump above my knee. When I showed it to a dermatologist, she unceremoniously told me to take off my trousers and lie down on her examination table. As she numbed the area and began to cut, I put my hands over my face. She said, "Am I hurting you?" No, I said. It was the shock. I knew nothing about melanoma except that it was particularly aggressive and lethal.

Follow-up surgery to remove more surrounding skin and to biopsy
a sentinel lymph node in my upper thigh (the most likely node to
which cells from my primary tumor would spread first) revealed no
further evidence of disease. The tumor's depth suggested that my
prospects were alarming enough: there was a 20 percent chance of
recurrence.

I was not yet ready to die, and I began to make decisions about
things I had avoided or neglected. I resolved to get divorced, something my then wife and I had been considering for years. The stress
of cancer is like a gale: it drives distant couples further apart and
compels already close ones to cling more tightly together.

In the next few years, I had periodic skin examinations and chest
X rays. Everything looked normal. Of course, anxiety lingered.

Metastasis

By 2000 I had gotten divorced and met Françoise, a theoretical
chemist, shortly after we had both entered the new world of online
dating. We became a devoted couple over the next three years.

As I got up from bed one night, I felt a kumquat-size lump in the
same lymph node bed that had been biopsied seven years before. I
sat back down heavily and whispered a curse, waking Françoise. She
wondered what was wrong—a nightmare, perhaps? I knew it was far
worse.

The lump was confirmed as melanoma a few days later. We were
stunned. Statistics suggested that my five-year survival chances had
just plummeted to 20 percent.

Everything suddenly became uncertain and threatening. My focus
changed. Concerns about world affairs, money, and social and professional status all receded. After a few days, Françoise said, "Jonathan, you have to take early retirement." I replied, "And we have to
get married." Again, delay made no sense. We quickly married a few
days before I had surgery to remove the entire lymph node bed.

For the next five years, my disease continued to spread very slowly. One oncologist said, "Either your immune system is very smart or your tumor is just very stupid." Nevertheless, I underwent two deeper surgeries in my lower right abdomen and joined two ineffective clinical trials. Another very promising drug trial targeting the common *BRAF* mutation was irrelevant in my case—tests showed that my tumors lacked that mutation.

Immunotherapy

By 2008 Françoise and I had retired to rural Connecticut, and I came under the care of Mario Sznol, leader of Yale University's Melanoma Clinical Research Program. After carefully reviewing my earlier scans and history, he shocked us with the news that the disease had already spread to my lungs. My melanoma had reached stage IV, and I had a median expected survival of eight months.

Dr. Sznol said that chemotherapy or further surgery was pointless; immunotherapy was my best remaining option. However, the two forms available at the time (alpha interferon and interleukin-2) had extremely low success rates. I was treated with both, and they had no apparent impact on my disease. They did, however, cause nasty side effects. Alpha interferon gave me chills and a bad rash. I felt exhausted and spent most of the day in bed. Interleukin-2 disoriented me and caused me to gain 30 pounds within a week. I ended up in the cardiac ward.

Fortunately, the effects were all quickly reversible. And Dr. Sznol said that immunotherapy drugs then in development offered great hope, particularly something called anti-PD-1 (the "PD" stands for programmed death). It had just begun clinical trials a short time before.

Unlike chemotherapy, which simply kills susceptible cells, the goal of immunotherapy is to boost the production of certain white blood cells (the T cells) that can then detect and kill tumors. The old immunotherapy strategy of giving patients high doses of the molecules (such as interleukin-2 and alpha interferon) that normally stimulate

T-cell production rarely worked because the immune system has its own brakes, or checkpoints, that prevent the accumulation of very high levels of these molecules. When the levels reach a certain point, the immune system shuts down its own production of the molecules.

In the 1980s, James P. Allison at the University of California, Berkeley, realized that a better strategy was to block or inhibit the checkpoints themselves, taking the normal brakes off the body's T-cell production. Almost 30 years after his group identified such a major checkpoint in mice (the CTLA-4 protein receptor), its blocking antibody finally gained approval from the Food and Drug Administration (FDA) for use in humans with advanced melanoma in 2011 (Bristol-Myers Squibb's anti-CTLA-4 antibody, ipilimumab).

Ipilimumab's journey to the market wasn't easy. Many melanoma patients anxiously followed the drug's slow path through clinical trials, which began in 2000. Because the drug acted differently from chemotherapy, it confused researchers and regulators. In many cases, tumors might initially grow rapidly before slowly melting away, and some unexpected side effects such as colitis could be particularly severe—even causing some trial patients to die. Early trials (managed by Medarex) failed to meet expectations, mainly because traditional chemotherapy goals (for example, measurable tumor reduction within a short time) were used for assessment.

The delays were frustrating and demoralizing. For support, Françoise suggested that I join the online forum of the Melanoma International Foundation (MIF). The forum helped patients in their searches for promising clinical trials. Nevertheless, my tumors were spreading, and most of the patients I came to know and care about on the forum died.

In 2010, I and other patients with advanced melanoma were able to get ipilimumab a few months before its FDA approval through an expanded access program. My side effects were manageable, and twelve weeks after I began treatment, scans showed clear signs that my tumors had begun to shrink.

Optimism suddenly returned in a rush—perhaps I would survive after all. However, I was not one of the truly fortunate 10 percent of patients who became completely tumor-free following ipilimumab treatment. After a year and a half, new tumors began to appear in my brain, lungs, intestines, and abdomen. Although I had no painful symptoms yet, the cancer was metastasizing throughout my body.

Anti-PD-1

My hope now centered on another immunotherapy checkpoint inhibitor, the anti-PD-1 drug that Dr. Sznol had mentioned to me years earlier. In 2008, Bristol-Myers Squibb had begun clinical trials for an anti-PD-1 drug that appeared to be more tolerable than ipilimumab and produce better survival rates. The initial clinical trial I tried to join was oversubscribed, and I was excluded from later ones either because I'd had a questionable biopsy for prostate cancer (like so many men my age) or because I'd had previous immunotherapy treatment.

My frustration and despair mounted. I and some other MIF members wrote and phoned Bristol-Myers Squibb executives to ask why the anti-PD-1 drug was not moving more quickly through trials. I also wrote top executives at the FDA and the National Cancer Institute, trying to speed up the drug's approval process—all to no avail.

My health continued to decline. The growing tumors now began to cause discomfort in my intestines, abdominal muscles, and lungs. I required almost weekly blood transfusions because of internal bleeding. I tried a second and third round of ipilimumab with modest effects and another experimental anti-PD-1 drug from a small Israeli biotechnology company. Nothing worked.

I began to accept my imminent death. I had lived the life I had desired. I had found my life's companion and confidante. I had repaired some frayed family relations. I had even lived to see a granddaughter born.

In April 2013, Catherine Poole of MIF suggested that I try a novel chemotherapy trial in Nashville, Tennessee. The trial drug was an antibody-drug conjugate, in which two molecules that bind preferentially to melanoma cells are linked to an especially toxic agent, auristatin. This reduced the drug's toxicity to other cells. I flew to Nashville for treatments periodically during the next 10 months. However, after I'd had a good response to the drug for seven months, the cancer recommenced its relentless advance.

A few months later, Poole told me that an expanded access program for Merck's competing anti-PD-1 drug (pembrolizumab) had just begun for advanced melanoma patients. I was able to join the trial and flew to the Mayo Clinic in Jacksonville, Florida, twice in May 2014 for infusions. By then I was too weak to walk through airports, and Françoise had to push me in a wheelchair.

Crisis and Recovery

I transferred my pembrolizumab treatment to Yale as soon as it was offered there, in June 2014. Tumors were intermittently blocking my small intestine, causing severe cramping and vomiting. An uncomfortable tube was inserted into my stomach via my nose. I was now in and out of emergency departments, taking opiates and hoping for a quick response to the drug. However, the blockages did not resolve themselves.

I was hospitalized, receiving nourishment via IV infusion only, and a second tube was inserted directly into my stomach. I had arrived at death's door. I had conversations with my family in anticipation of the end. One way or another, I was prepared to move on.

I was offered abdominal surgery to remove the obstructing tumors in my intestines. However, the attending surgeon was hesitant because other tumors would remain and grow. Another attending physician was clearly pessimistic. But Dr. Sznol said that there was a real chance the drug could eliminate the remaining disease after the surgery. Although things might "go the other way," he said, there was the potential for me to regain a normal life. That was a prospect we couldn't refuse.

The operation was unexpectedly rough. When the surgical team opened my abdomen, my intestines popped out onto my belly from the accumulated pressure. My intestine had perforated en route to the operating room and was starting to leak stool. If the team had waited a few hours longer, I would have died from an infection. They removed almost a yard of intestine and created an ileostomy—a diversion of my small intestine through an opening in my abdominal wall, bypassing my colon.

I awoke in excruciating pain and was distraught when they told me how the operation had gone. I told the surgical team I didn't want to live. Everyone suddenly became quiet.

The surgeon leaned over me and said, "Dr. Friedlaender, you will be out of most of the discomfort and off the opiates in a couple of days. The tubes to your stomach will come out, the IV nutrition will stop, and very soon you'll be able to eat again. In two weeks you should be able to go home as you've wanted so badly." It was also possible that the ileostomy would be reversible in time.

Françoise reminded me that it would take another month to know if the anti-PD-1 drug was working and said that I should not lose hope. This calmed me.

My recovery at home was difficult. I was very weak after almost six weeks in the hospital. Françoise became my constant nurse. I slowly regained my strength and began to take care of myself. My next scans showed that I was responding to the drug, and the prospect of imminent death immediately receded. The doctors were now all smiles. The surgery plus the immunotherapy had come in the very nick of time.

Two years after my crisis, I have one remaining pea-size tumor in my armpit. It will probably continue to shrivel away. I just stopped taking the anti-PD-1 drug last month. If the disease recurs, I could resume immunotherapy treatment or some combination of therapies. When I die, Dr. Sznol says, it will be from something besides this horrible disease that I have come to know so intimately.

Reforming Clinical Trials

During this 20-year journey, I necessarily learned a good deal about drug development and approvals. I also became an FDA patient representative, which taught me even more. The number of new drugs approved by the FDA has been increasing in the past three years, and 51 were approved in 2015—the highest number since 1950.

Immunotherapy drugs are among the greatest recent successes. The approved combination therapy of an anti-PD-1 drug and ipilimumab for advanced melanoma has had "stunning" effects, according to Dr. Harriet Kluger of Yale University. Immunotherapy drugs have been approved or are in trials for over 30 other solid tumor malignancies. Cancers of the kidney, bladder, and lung, as well as refractory Hodgkin's lymphoma, have all been shown to respond to anti-PD-1 drugs at varying but clinically significant rates.

Although things are beginning to change, the drug approval process has been unnecessarily slow. During my long illness, I felt akin to the HIV/AIDS patients of 30 years ago, when exciting protease inhibitors were in development but not yet widely available. When an especially promising treatment is identified, we have to find acceptable ways to facilitate its approval and allow earlier access to it for people who are critically ill.

Faced with imminent death, informed patients have the right to risk their lives by taking a promising but unproven drug, just as they have the right to decide when to terminate further treatment. Withholding drugs in such situations is unethical and paternalistic, even if it may violate the physician's Hippocratic oath to "first, do no harm." There is certainly no excuse for trial designs that have placebo or standard treatment arms without a timely crossover provision for ultimate access to the trial drug.

After a great deal of criticism, the FDA does now recognize that when a drug shows early evidence of superiority, a small and relatively short trial with appropriately designed goals (such as surrogate endpoints instead of mortality rates) could support a provisional approval. This means waiving the randomized double-blind final trial that has been the "gold standard" since the thalidomide scandal over 50 years ago. Such trials have become a cumbersome multibillion-dollar enterprise.

According to the FDA, in fiscal year 2014 two-thirds of the newly approved drugs had been granted some kind of accelerated review. The "breakthrough therapy" designation, initiated in 2012, allowed Merck's anti-PD-1 drug to go through its clinical trials and win FDA approval in three years (2011–14). This saved the lives of many critically ill patients, including me.

Medicines approved in this way are necessarily monitored closely afterward for undiscovered risks and interactions. This is really the way it should be for all drugs: first achieving provisional approval by satisfying a set of FDA-dictated goals in a restricted population, and then having close postapproval monitoring in a large clinical setting. Parallel efforts to speed up and humanize the drug approval process are also under way in the European Medicines Agency's "adaptive licensing" pilot project.

Reining In Drug Costs

I was amazed by the prices of new drugs. The largest pharmaceutical companies are certainly benefiting handsomely. Their net profitability consistently ranks among the highest of the major industrial sectors, according to BBC News, and pharmaceutical research and development spending, while certainly large, is generally less than spending on marketing and advertising, as the World Health Organization has noted. Prices in the United States are particularly high: in a 2004 article in the *New York Review of Books*, Marcia Angell referred to the United States as the primary prescription drug "profit center."

Beginning with their testimony in the 1959–62 hearings of the US Senate Subcommittee on Antitrust and Monopoly investigating drug costs, chaired by Sen. Estes Kefauver (D-TN), pharmaceutical companies have justified the high prices of prescription drugs because of their development costs, which are linked to especially long development times and high failure rates. The latest controversial estimate from the Tufts Center for the Study of Drug Development, an industry-supported source, for the cost of the successful development of a new drug is $2.6 billion. However, the CEO of GlaxoSmithKline has called this figure a myth, and Médecins Sans Frontières suggests that more realistic figures might be less than one-tenth of that number.

Newer value-based rationales for high drug prices also appear problematic, as it is very hard to calculate the worth of a drug—especially just after approval. For example, value-pricing a drug such as an anti-PD-1 drug should mean a comparatively high price for treating melanoma but a much lower one for treating lung cancer, where it is less effective. Drug prices clearly are not dictated by these circumstances. Instead, after reviewing the arguments surrounding drug pricing, a hundred experts on chronic myeloid leukemia concluded in a May 2013 article in *Blood*, "Of the many complex factors involved, price often seems to follow a simple formula: start with the price for the most recent similar drug on the market and price the new one within 10% to 20% of that price (usually higher)."

Drug companies simply charge what they think the market will bear.

The price of a drug can vary dramatically not only from one country to another but from patient to patient. The negotiated price to my insurer of each infusion of pembrolizumab I received was $9,000, or $153,000 for 17 infusions during a year (the list, or off-the-shelf, price for one infusion was $52,000). However, the price for a friend who has different health insurance but received identical treatment was four times as much—about $600,000 per year. The difference is apparently because my insurer's negotiating group was bigger and had more leverage than that of my friend's insurer.

A Survivor's Perspective

I have been incredibly fortunate. My disease was especially indolent. I was able to retire early and look for promising clinical trials. I certainly could not have survived without the continuing support of my wife, Françoise. I was treated in an outstanding university teaching hospital that had expertise in immunotherapy, and I had comprehensive health insurance. My multiple surgeries, plus the expensive drug treatments, were enough to bankrupt almost anyone without coverage. My biggest out-of-pocket expense was commuting to Nashville for 10 months, which totaled $8,000.

During the long struggle, I experienced both remarkable and distressing aspects of the US health care system. I am trying as best I can to contribute to its correction, improvement, and humanization. Everything has changed in my life. There is much to appreciate and savor, and much more to do.

A Black Alzheimer's Patient Wants to Be Part of the Cure

A daughter gets her mother into a clinical trial for an Alzheimer's drug, with few other black patients enrolled.

Katti Gray

At her thirty-third appearance as Subject 16019 in a clinical trial of an experimental drug she hoped would fix "this little problem with my memory," Sandra Brannon sank into a medical exam room's recliner and waited.

"What's the date again?" Sandra asked me. I had escorted her to a wing at Bellevue Hospital Center in Manhattan, where NYU Lan-

Volume 36, Number 6. June 2017.

gone Medical Center was conducting the trial—one of 210 institutions worldwide doing so. As a family friend, I was standing in for Sandra's only child and chief caregiver, Monica Montgomery. Thirty-five-year-old Monica was a globetrotter and had business elsewhere that morning.

"November eighteenth," I answered.

I'd responded to the same question from Sandra four times during our 27-minute ride from a Brooklyn Bridge subway station to Bellevue.

"Right. Got it." Sandra scribbled my reply on her cheat sheet as a nurse bounded through the door to prep her for her monthly intravenous infusion of the experimental drug solanezumab, which Eli Lilly developed to target mild cognitive impairment caused by Alzheimer's.

"How was your commute here?" the nurse began.

Sandra had been diagnosed with Alzheimer's in 2011, at the age of 64. She was 69 on that day at Bellevue. Sandra's mother had died of the incurable degenerative disease in March 2004 at the age of 83, about seven years after her diagnosis.

"Any changes in your health since the last time we saw you?" the nurse continued, probing Sandra. "You know what today is?"

Sandra cheerfully wiggled and snapped her fingers. She let out a blip of laughter and grinned.

"The third of May?" She hesitated, looked at the nurse's raised eyebrows, and realized she'd gotten it wrong. "No. Ummm—oh, yes, it's November eighteenth, Friday."

"You looked at your pad, huh?" the nurse said, smiling and gently patting Sandra's hand. She pushed two plastic water-cooler cups toward her: "You're dehydrated, and we can't get the needle into your vein easily when you're dehydrated. Drink this."

That cheat sheet of scribbled notes and details had become Sandra's brace and comfort during visits to that special NYU Langone wing at Bellevue. It was ground zero in her quest for something—anything—to slow her dementia. As a black woman, she played a critical role in the trial, and not just because of her own plight: blacks and Latinos are diagnosed with Alzheimer's more often than whites. Yet during those many visits to that wing, Sandra seemed to be the only black patient present. Ever.

"From the beginning of this," Monica told me, "I'd see lots of little white ladies lovingly leading their girlfriends into the office and asking questions: 'I hear you have a clinical trial for Alzheimer's? We want to get in that.' But hardly ever—if ever—did I see others of us, black people, there signing up for the same thing."

When Eli Lilly reported preliminary results of the trial in December 2016, the data told a similar story: 90.8 percent of the trial participants who reported their race were white, 1.7 percent were black.

Getting into the Trial

Sandra grew up in Washington, DC, the child of a schoolteacher and a preacher, and she moved to New York straight out of high school to study art at the Pratt Institute. I'd met her and Monica more than 20 years earlier at Emmanuel Baptist Church in Brooklyn. At the time, Monica was active in the church's Teen Canteen group, Sandra was a trustee, and I did double duty as a choir member and newsletter editor.

At the start of our surrogate kinship, Sandra was assistant principal at a high school. She'd gone into education after being a graphic designer at the *New York Times* and CBS News. She switched careers as computer-made illustrations were supplanting the pen-and-pencil renderings that she preferred. Plus, an educator's work hours were more suited to raising a child during a rocky marriage. She and her husband, a college professor, divorced when Monica was a teenager. That was back when Sandra, voluble and vibrant, commanded a room, weighing in on any discussion and perhaps, to liven things up, peppering the conversation with cuss words.

Monica was living in DC when she first noticed Sandra's lapses. Sandra had driven there to visit her, but on her way back to New York, she called Monica to ask what highway she was supposed to take.

Over time, Sandra started repeating herself and misplacing things. "She was having these small accidents," Monica says. "Bumping a street sign with her car. Losing her keys, wallet. It was scary, nerve-racking . . . and I instantly knew what it was."

Years earlier, Monica had been involved, hands-on, in her grandmother's 24-hour care at the end of her life. Eventually, home health aides were hired as well.

"I knew this thing ran in families," Monica says. "I felt this disappointment and dread, and rugged resignation."

Monica is an arts activist and museum curator who has lectured internationally and been an adjunct professor at Harvard University. Like her mom, she is charismatic, whip-smart, and a life-of-the-party type. Like her mom, she can be no-nonsense and resolute. Her resolve would serve her well after her mom was diagnosed.

An internist in a private practice, who was also black, had diagnosed Sandra but offered little in the way of treatment options. Instead, the physician recommended that Sandra do crossword puzzles and that the family hope for the best. After Monica's repeated requests, the doctor finally prescribed Aricept, a treatment for mild-to-moderate Alzheimer's symptoms.

Monica was living in Philadelphia then. She emptied her rental and moved back to her mom's Brooklyn apartment. As she researched Alzheimer's and searched for physicians lauded for their work on the disease, she also conferred with a dear friend, a geriatric social worker, about how to move forward. In the fall of 2013, Monica chose a neurologist at NYU Langone Health's Center for Cognitive Neurology to treat her mother and began discussing how to enroll her in a clinical trial.

"Actually getting her into the trial was an uphill battle," Monica says.

They needed a letter from Sandra's diagnosing physician, but she ignored Monica's pleas for assistance.

"At a certain point I just rolled in there and, without causing a scene, said 'My mom is deteriorating,'" Monica remembers.

She also wrote a pointed letter to the Center for Cognitive Neurology. She was frustrated after too many delays and *we'll see*'s.

In the fall of 2014, Sandra joined what ultimately were the 2,129 patients in Eli Lilly's trial of solanezumab at those 210 sites in the United States, Canada, Australia, Japan, and Europe. Sandra was notified in fall 2015 that she was being infused with solanezumab and not the trial's placebo drug.

Sandra's optimism spiked.

Minorities in Clinical Trials

In 1994 the National Institutes of Health (NIH) mandated that participants' enrollment in NIH-approved clinical trials reflect the nation's racial makeup and gender breakdown.

Whites accounted for 61.6 percent of the US population in July 2015, according to the most recent census data. Census analysts project that share to dip to 44 percent by 2060 if current trends hold. And in 2020 more than half of the nation's children up to age 18 are projected to be people of color, the Census Bureau says.

According to a 2013 NIH report, minorities accounted for 36.5 percent of the 17.6 million participants in NIH-registered clinical trials of drugs and other medical interventions in fiscal year 2012.

But researchers in the EMPaCT Consortium, which provides training to medical professionals and community organizations on the mechanics of clinical trials in a bid to increase minority participation in trials, estimate the share of minority participants in NIH-registered clinical trials to be less than 10 percent. Depending on the disease targeted by a trial, that rate could be even lower. A study published in *Cancer* in April 2014 concluded that fewer than 2 percent of National Cancer Institute clinical trials focused primarily on any minority population.

The percentage of minorities in clinical trials conducted by drug manufacturers—which now carry out the vast majority of drug trials—is more difficult to pin down. According to Nathaniel Stinson, a medical doctor who heads the Division of Scientific Programs at the National Institute on Minority Health and Health Disparities, companies often don't disclose much—if any—information about the race of participants or other aspects of their trials until the trials are over.

"At that point, everything, regrettably, is after the fact," he says.

Increasing Minority Enrollment

Given the nation's changing demographics, it's neither good health policy nor good business to be developing drugs and possible cures that are tested in only a subset of the population, says Willie Deese, who retired in June 2016 as executive vice president at Merck. Months after retiring, he earmarked part of a $1 million gift to the North Carolina Agricultural and Technical State University in Greensboro—a historically black college and Deese's alma mater—for its groundbreaking Center for Outreach in Alzheimer's, Aging and Community Health. In addition to collecting and studying the DNA of black patients with Alzheimer's, the center provides support services for such patients and their caregivers and educates blacks about scientific research.

Deese, whose mother has Alzheimer's, says there's a growing recognition within the black community that its members can't be absent from clinical trials and expect medicine to work as well for them as it does for other populations.

"We have to be included," he says. "Enlightened companies are ensuring that that's taking place today."

Raegan Durant, an internist and professor at the University of Alabama at Birmingham, believes that scientists and policy makers are far more aware today of the critical need for a diversity of clinical trial participants than they were when the NIH issued its mandate. But the challenge is figuring out how best to achieve a representative mix and to keep the recruitment of minority volunteers from being an afterthought.

"There must be a shared power," he says, "between science and laypeople."

The almost-four-year-old Mississippi State Department of Health's Community Research Fellows Training Program is considered one leading model of change. It schools community members in how trials work and partners with grassroots organizations that directors of the fellows project view as deeply invested in public health and wellness. It's creating a community-clinician conversation about trials in the hope, among others, of keeping doctors from mentioning clinical trial enrollment opportunities at the moment when they deliver a dire medical diagnosis. That might be the least opportune time to raise the possibility of joining a trial.

Thus far, some of the more than 50 graduates of the intensive four-months-long training program have gone on to sit on clinical trial institutional review boards in Mississippi and to win grants for public health initiatives.

Still, as more minorities express interest in enrolling in clinical trials, there are some looming questions and challenges: How can medical science and the culture surrounding trials be demystified? Should clinical trials continue to exclude, as they generally do, patients with comorbidities—especially given the disproportionate percentage of minorities with more than one illness?

"That's the million-dollar question," says Michelle Martin, a preventive medicine professor and researcher who was hired by the University of Tennessee Health Science Center in 2016 to help shape its research programs.

"It probably does matter in some cases," Martin tells me. "But there has been a movement toward more pragmatic trials where the inclusion-exclusion criteria are a little broader."

Whether trials accommodate the everyday circumstances of participants is another key concern. What of the added costs of taking time away from a job to keep a spate of clinical trial appointments? What of a participant's childcare or eldercare needs? Who'll put gas in the tank or cover public transit costs so participants can get to trial sites?

Too often patients and caregivers are solving those problems on their own and doing all the legwork needed to get into clinical trials they hope will benefit their health, says Jennifer Wenzel, a professor at Johns Hopkins University's School of Nursing and School of Medicine and an EMPaCT researcher and advocate. It's an unfair burden, she says.

Some patient navigators specializing in clinical trials have helped trial participants of color stick with their experimental treatments. The navigators function as patient advocates. They serve as liaisons between patients and their physicians and trial researchers. They whisk away tears. They explain things. They cheer on participants and have helped ensure that patients stay on board until the trial ends. Yet navigators are not spread across the entire clinical trial system, and some health systems that do have them struggle with how to compensate them for their time and effort.

Meanwhile, experts say that private physicians, no matter the many demands on their time at work, must do more to change the racial makeup of trials. Referrals to trials may be more common at university-run medical centers, where staff members know about on-campus research and help funnel patients to those researchers. Unfortunately, not every doctor has this access or will make the effort.

Epilogue

In November 2016, Eli Lilly reported that solanezumab had no effect on people with mild Alzheimer's symptoms and began winding down the trial. Monica forwarded the emails from the NYU researchers to me. She and her mother were crushed by the drug's failings. Monica tried not to show her mother the fullness of her disappointment and anger, afraid they would rub off. They decided that Sandra's thirty-fourth appointment at Bellevue would be her last, though she had been given the option to make more visits to the clinic.

Monica requested all of her mother's clinical trial files, the stuff in the black vinyl binder that nurses annotated during Sandra's monthly visits. For being a trial volunteer, Sandra had gotten a $40 monthly stipend and extravigilant checks of her weight loss, blood pressure, cholesterol level, and assorted physiological markers. Monica wanted those notations.

"I want a written report of their findings and her progress, if she made any," she tells me. "I just want more insight into my mom's health."

Today Sandra is no longer avidly reading the *New York Times*. She does head to a senior citizen center several afternoons a week, but only if Monica lists the landmarks along the way for her, a new kind of crutch.

For 14 consecutive days this March, Sandra phoned the doorman of her high-rise co-op apartment building for instructions on using the elevator that had ferried her for four decades.

"She just stands in front of it at times, totally bewildered," Monica says.

Monica and the home health aide decided that Sandra should no longer light the stove to cook anything. She has grudgingly surrendered her driver's license and the keys to her Toyota. Except for sporadic engagement with a handful of friends, she is more isolated than ever.

Yet when I talk to her after the clinical trial ended, Sandra sounds pretty chipper, all things considered. She once told me that she veers toward joy, no matter what life throws at her.

"Thank you," she tells me, "for being my balm in Gilead."

An emotion I cannot name rears up in me. My eyes tear.

"You're my jewel and joy," I say. "Let's get our nails done and go to lunch soon."

"Absolutely," she says. "And you never know. The drug they were giving me might kick in."

Monica shares her mother's cautious optimism.

"We still hope, somehow, that all of this will lead to a cure," she says. "We can feel like my mom was a part of that."

3

Patient-Centered Care

- "Nothing Is Broken": For an Injured Doctor, Quality-Focused Care Misses the Mark *Charlotte Yeh*

- The Battle of the Bundle: Lessons from My Mother's Partial Hip Replacement *Timothy Hoff*

- Even in an Emergency, Doctors Must Make Informed Consent an Informed Choice *Cindy Brach*

"Nothing Is Broken"

For an Injured Doctor, Quality-Focused Care Misses the Mark

When a physician winds up in the emergency department, providers put quality metrics and testing before her actual needs.

Charlotte Yeh

It was just after six o'clock in the evening on Wednesday, December 7, 2011—Pearl Harbor Day—when I left my organization's Washington, DC, office to meet a colleague for dinner. It was dark and rainy, and I had one more intersection to cross to get to the restaurant. I was about a third of the way across the intersection when I heard a loud "thump" and felt a sharp pain squarely in my backside. A dialogue unfolded in my head: "Wow! I wonder what that was . . . I think it was me. No, I don't think it was me. Wait . . . I think I just got hit by a car! But there's no way!" Before I could even make sense of the situation, I had flown through the air and landed on the street.

"Are you OK?" a man frantically asked me. I was so stunned that I said nothing—highly unusual for me. The man called for an ambulance. I feared I might be run over, lying there where drivers couldn't see me. Two other men approached, keen on moving me out of the street. But as an emergency physician, I knew that trauma training tells us never to move victims. You're supposed to splint a victim where she lies so as not to injure her back or neck. But I also remembered that personal safety comes first. In those fleeting moments lying there on the pavement, I debated whether to stay where I was and risk being run over or allow myself to be moved and risk further injury. I chose personal safety. I tried to mentally assess the damage to my neck and back and asked the two men to get me off the street.

Volume 33, Number 6. June 2014.

They carried me through the pouring rain into a nearby restaurant, where I waited for the ambulance. When the EMTs arrived, they placed a C-collar around my neck and positioned me on a backboard for the short ride to the hospital, a Level I trauma center.

I was wheeled into the hospital's ambulance entrance, where the triage nurse met me and confirmed that I could speak English. An EMT briefed the nurse, noting that I had been hit by a car.

"Where were you sitting?" the nurse asked.

"I wasn't sitting in a car," I said.

"Were you in the passenger seat or the driver's seat?" she continued.

"No, I wasn't sitting in a car," I said. "I was walking across the street."

It took several rounds of back-and-forth before she understood that I was in an "auto-ped" accident, as they call it in emergency department (ED) lingo. Perhaps the nurse thought I looked too "whole" for this to be true.

The admitting ED team scurried me into an examination room, where they asked if I was having any pain. It seemed an incongruous question, seeing as a car had just plowed into me. Yes, I was in considerable pain, I told them. They inserted an IV, and morphine began to flow.

A doctor came in and commenced the "primary survey," an initial exam to detect any risk of life- or limb-threatening emergencies. Then came a brief evaluation to ensure that I could come out of the C-collar and off the backboard, a visual inspection for external bleeding or misaligned bones, and an assurance that my heart and lungs were functioning normally. I told the doctor that I had severe pain in my knee and backside. "OK, we're going to need a CT [computed tomography] of the abdomen, CT of the pelvis, and X-rays of the chest," she said. Something didn't seem right to me. Wasn't she going to examine my knee and backside?

When the tests were completed, I was wheeled out of the exam room, still flat on my back. By this time, roughly three hours after the accident, the ED was chaotically busy and all of the rooms were filled, so I was parked in the hallway. A new round of clinicians—presumably the admitting trauma team, although I wasn't sure—stopped by my stretcher. "Well, everything looks fine on your tests," the head clinician informed me. "There's a little bleeding in the muscle around your hip area. We just don't know if that's going to continue, so we want to watch it. We're going to admit you." I gasped. I was still in denial that I had any serious injuries.

An inpatient bed wasn't available yet, so I would be "boarded" in the hallway until one opened up.

I lay there on my gurney all night—nearly 15 hours—with my work BlackBerry, my personal cell phone, and a morphine drip, watching the bustle of hospital traffic around me. Several times during the night, my blood pressure was taken. When the pain returned every two or three hours, I caught the eye of hassled staff members and had them tell the nurse, who would come by to give me a quick infusion of morphine.

Having spent many years serving in EDs as an emergency physician, I took comfort in being left in the hallway. It meant that I was OK, that the hospital staff wasn't so worried about me. As a patient, though, I felt alone. I was struck by the demeanor of some hospital staff who rushed by. It seemed as if they were deliberately avoiding eye contact with any of us poor souls waiting in the hallway, lest they be interrupted and asked for help. I wanted contact. Even after assuring my long-distance daughters by phone that I was OK, I wanted someone present, looking out for me.

Good to Go?

In the morning the day crew appeared, taking over from the night crew. Residents went from gurney to gurney, sorting out patient dispositions. Around this time, the day crew learned that I was an emergency physician and, out of deference and consideration, they moved me out of the hallway into a private room, assuming this is what I would want. The private room was darkened so I could sleep, and the door was shut. Now, instead of feeling safe in the controlled chaos of the corridor, I felt abandoned, clutching my nurse call button, a lifeline to the world.

A new admitting trauma team stopped by later in the day to review my case. Because I had been stable all night and no major injuries had turned up on the CT scans, they decided I was ready for discharge. "Nothing is broken; you can go home now," said one of the team members.

I was stunned. I was still in excruciating viselike pain, and my knee and backside still hadn't been checked. The "good patient" in me wanted to please the doctor and saunter out of the room, but the real person in me was scared. I told the team that I wasn't able to walk after the accident and wasn't sure I could walk now. I was traveling on business and staying alone in a hotel room, so I might not be able to care for myself, I said. Again, they told me: "Nothing is broken, so you can walk."

Even though no one examined my swollen right knee or left hip area to determine the extent of my injuries beyond broken bones, I knew that serious ligament or cartilage injuries could be sustained without broken bones. No one had talked with me about whether I would be able to function safely at home or about follow-up care either.

But the "good patient" won over, so with trepidation, I said I was happy to go home. "Do you think I'll be OK at the hotel?" I said. "My knee is swollen, and I'm not sure I can walk on it."

"We'll just send in physical therapy to get you up and walking," the resident said.

A short time later, the physical therapy staff came in and looked me over. "We're supposed to get you up?" one of them asked. They attempted to stand me up, and I nearly crumpled to the floor. I couldn't support my weight, let alone walk. They helped me back onto the gurney and then left the room to go brief the admitting team.

The resident returned. "There's no medical reason to admit you," he said, "but if you can't walk, we'll just have to." The "good patient" in me felt embarrassed that somehow I had failed the "test" and was now an unnecessary admission, maybe taking the place of someone who needed the bed more than I did.

Diagnosis, Piece by Piece

The resident's comment struck me as callous, as if addressing my basic need to function and recover after the accident had nothing to do with the care he and his colleagues were there to provide. The team returned a bit later to tell me that a bed had opened up—in the maternity ward.

On that first day in the maternity ward, nurses came in and out as I asked, over and over it seemed, "Is anyone going to look at my knee?" By the end of the day, an orthopedic consultant appeared. He determined that I had a medial collateral ligament tear and recommended putting me in a splint and getting a formal magnetic resonance imaging (MRI) when I returned home to Boston. Finally, I had a partial diagnosis.

During that first day as an inpatient, I experienced increasing lower abdominal pain and told the staff a few times. I suspected a catheter malfunction. "Something feels wrong," I said. "Is my catheter working? My lower abdomen hurts, and the catheter doesn't feel right." I was told that catheters are irritating and always make you feel like you have to urinate. Each time I mentioned it, the bag was checked, the presence of urine was confirmed, and I was assured that the catheter was working. It wasn't until six hours later when the admitting team came by that they pulled back my sheets and exclaimed, "Did you know your catheter fell out?" as though it was my fault for not "telling the staff" or checking myself.

Over the next several hours, the piecemeal evaluation continued. That night, I began to experience numbness and tingling in my leg and my hip. I knew these were neurological symptoms and something wasn't right. Three times doctors or nurses came through, and each time I explained my concerns but was not evaluated. It wasn't until 24 hours later, during the night of my second day of hospitalization, that I had a neurological exam revealing contusion of both the sciatic and the gluteal nerves.

On my third day in the hospital, someone asked if the admitting trauma team had done a history and physical, standard procedure following the initial primary and secondary surveys. They had not. A resident then performed a "tertiary" exam—essentially, a repeat history and physical examination—although he and I both knew the prior exams had been incomplete.

By morning rounds on my fourth day in the hospital, I was both medically and functionally stable, able to ambulate cautiously with assistance and a walker. I insisted on being transferred to a rehabilitation facility near my home in Boston.

The Art of Care

Nearly two years after my accident, after extensive rehabilitation, I am still limping and walking with a cane. I have had to adjust my daily routines. I still need wheelchair assistance at airports and still struggle with my balance on ramps and uneven ground. It is a challenge to put away bath towels on an upper shelf without tipping over. I still can't ride a bike or hike. Even swinging open a door is problematic because I can't fully brace myself against the weight of the door.

The most dispiriting consequence of all, though, is the loss of independence. Every choice I make each day about where I go requires careful advance planning: What's the terrain? Will I need to ask for help? How long will it take for assistance to arrive? I depend on others now.

As a medical professional who became an accident victim and then a trauma patient, I was a participant-observer in emergency care, with a big-picture window into how well our health care system does or doesn't work. There's just something about being boarded on a gurney in a hospital hallway for 15 hours that gets one thinking about paradigm shifts.

In my case, I was struck by the uneven nature of my care, marked by an overreliance on testing and a narrow focus on limited quality metrics such as pain management or catheter care processes. Looking back, I believe that this approach fostered an inattention to my overall well-being. Instead of feeling like a connected patient at the center of care, I felt processed and disengaged. This is disconcerting, especially at a time when patient-centered care—that is, care delivered *with* me, not *to* me or *for* me—is becoming the new normal.

The Hippocratic oath, the medical profession's ethical creed, reads: "I will prescribe regimens for the good of my patients according to my ability and my judgment and never do harm to anyone." This vow compels physicians to heed both the "science" and the "art" of medicine. The science often lies in defining the treatment regimens. The art lies in understanding what matters personally to the patient.

Even in an ideal world, this would be a high bar to clear. Despite some national consensus on quality metrics, we have continued struggling to measure "the good of the patient." Still, quality metrics cannot alone advance the good of the patient. Focusing on clinical measures in particular is not enough as long as other measures that focus on patient-desired outcomes are ignored. If we don't understand what patients' expectations are, we can't engage patients effectively in their care.

Through my experience as a patient, I observed a bias in what the metrics track: toward the clinical and away from the personal. To help restore this balance and reassert the art of care, I see three areas that the medical community should address.

Beware the Culture of Testing

When a test, such as a CT scan or a blood exam, is the centerpiece of care strategies, patient care can be compromised. As medicine and technology evolve, we may have become victims of our own success. We have become test-happy and technology-powered. These tools may provide us with good data *on* the patient, but this doesn't mean we're serving the good *of* the patient.

In my case, test-based care, while absolutely necessary, could have been balanced with a better understanding of me as a person and what mattered to me.

The unintended consequence of our current approach is that the clinical measure can become more important than the patient. I am afraid that as a result, we may be training a new generation of practitioners to equate high-quality care with conducting a test. Instead of having the test be used to discover new information about the patient, it is being used to define if one even is a patient.

Personalizing Care

After I'd spent four days in the hospital, it dawned on me that not once had anybody come by to ask how I was doing, what I needed, what I wanted, or whether I had any concerns. I then understood something that my own patients had been telling me all the time: They don't feel *engaged* in their own care. There is nothing personal about it.

Weeks after my accident, I began rehabilitation treatment at a hospital in Massachusetts to work on activities of daily living, such as getting out of bed, using a walker, preparing meals in the kitchen, getting in and out of the car, putting socks on, taking a shower, and getting up and down the stairs. The art of care promised by the Hippocratic oath flickered back to life. Here, personalized patient care was the rule, not the exception. I saw staff treating every patient with dignity and respect and listening to what mattered to them.

Each member of the rehabilitation team asked me what "my goal" was—a simple enough inquiry. I told them it was to be able to go up and down the stairs in my house. No one ever asked me this during my acute hospitalization.

During my rehabilitation stay, I witnessed pure encouragement and compassion. Staff appreciated the patient's current capacities, physical and emotional, and showed a sophisticated understanding of the gradations of care and recovery. Care becomes personal when dignity is established, regardless of the setting.

Patient-Reported Outcomes

Patient-reported outcomes are a vital piece of the puzzle and are often overlooked because of institutional inertia or culture. In my case over those first four days, the management of my reported pain was perfect, a 10 out of 10—but it was the exception. Despite my requests for information and attention, it took a piecemeal evaluation over four days to sort out and diagnose the full damage to my body. My reports about my own condition did not seem to matter to anyone else.

Patient-reported outcomes currently in development, such as asking for the patient perspective ("what do you want," "what are your fears," "what matters to you") and equalizing the patient-provider dialogue, create shared partnership in the outcomes and might have made a difference in my care. Going forward, quality metrics should give more weight to patient-reported outcomes if we want to truly assess care more effectively. As my experience suggests, we're not quite there yet.

The "North Star" of Care

If I resolved anything on my care journey, it is that the "North Star" guiding all care must be providers using any means possible to know the patient, hear the patient, and respond to what matters to the patient. It should make no difference where you practice; any provider can do this. Emergency departments can't hide behind the excuses of "we're too busy" or "it's too chaotic" to avoid connecting with every patient.

It is time to frame a new paradigm of care, a consumer-driven approach that concentrates attention on the art of medicine. This might begin with a reinvigorated focus on patient-centered care and mastering the skills of listening, empathy, and patient partnership.

The Oath of Maimonides, another code for the medical calling, offers a hopeful note about the physician: "Today he can discover his errors of yesterday, and tomorrow he can obtain a new light on what he thinks himself sure of today." Should this wisdom prevail, the next generation of quality measurement may strike that elusive balance between the clinical and the personal, and the good of the patient will always guide the care we deliver.

The Battle of the Bundle

Lessons from My Mother's Partial Hip Replacement

For one family, Medicare's bundled payment program felt more like a health care assembly line than coordinated care.

Timothy Hoff

Listening in on the phone—me three hours away at work in Boston and my siblings sitting in a rehabilitation facility outside of New York City—I could feel the anger rising in my throat. I was fed up. So were they. A week after having a partial hip replacement, our 90-year-old mother with dementia was being talked about as if she were some willfully noncompliant patient, slowing down her own rehabilitation for some self-interested purpose only she knew about. This is wrong, I thought. My mother is scared and hurt, and she needs to be embraced by the health care system right now, not run through it as if she were just like everyone else. So I spoke up for her, because she could not.

My mother is like a lot of people her age, yet she's also different. She's unique in many ways, at least to us. A human spitfire her entire life, she was born and raised on the streets of New York City, the second-youngest of six children of Irish immigrants. She and my father raised my four siblings and me in challenging living circumstances (the Bronx in the 1970s), spending their hard-earned dollars to give us a good education and a roof over our heads. The apartment where I grew up was crowded yet warm and loving. My mother could give you a lot of grief, but at the same time she'd go all out to protect you from harm. I still remember how she picked me up for lunch every day at one point in grammar school so I could eat at home in peace and not have to deal with the increasingly mean streets of the school playground. That was her.

Volume 36, Number 8. August 2017.

But she's lived a long time, and things happen to people who live a long time—most of them not good. She was healthy most of her life, but the past several years have been increasingly unkind. First came the onset of dementia, a terrible disease that slowly guts a person's personality and awareness. With the dementia came the inevitable slowdown in locomotion activity: She was increasingly holed up in a tiny apartment just north of New York City that she shared with my brother, without whose caregiving she would have ended up in a nursing home several years ago. But she spent more and more time sitting in the recliner, staring at the television, and sleeping. Still, our family thought that was better than being in an institutional setting.

Finally, and somewhat inevitably, the fall came. My mother's low bone density, dementia fog, and difficulty getting up from her chair conspired to make it happen. With a part-time home health aide and my brother living at home, the moments when my mother was left alone had become increasingly rare. But during one of those moments, she tried to get out of her chair and tripped. Up to that moment, it had been a day for her like any other from the past year or so. Lots of sitting, lots of dozing, lots of calls to my brother. A neighbor keeping tabs on her heard her calls for help and contacted my brother at work. He then called our sister, who went over to the apartment to find our mother on the floor. An ambulance arrived shortly afterward to take her to a local community hospital's emergency room.

She had fractured her left hip, the dreaded injury that—alongside damaged knees—hits the elderly hard and eats up so many Medicare inpatient dollars, often through partial or full joint replacements. When I got the call from my brother that he was at the emergency room with her, her future came clearly into focus: That day would be her last sitting in their small apartment, having some degree of independence. She was about to become dependent on a fragmented, competitive system of health care payers and delivery organizations. She would traverse the modern elderly person's trail of tears: from emergency room to hospital bed to operating room to rehabilitation hospital to nursing home. With luck she would avoid the intensive care unit (ICU). As for me, I would have to watch the fireball of my youth and adulthood reduced to a passive passenger on the cold, loud train to Long-Term Careville.

Entering the Assembly Line

I've worked in, studied, and taught health care as an administrator, consultant, and university-based academic for the past 30 years, so I knew more than the rest of my family did about the maze of complexity, uncertainty, and risk that my mother was entering. Older folks, already debilitated by a significant injury, often endured a steady drip of secondary morbidities in hospitals and rehabilitation facilities, such as infections and pressure sores. And the clinical interventions meant to prevent, slow, or stop those morbidities often compromised the patients' immune systems and set them up for something even worse down the road (pneumonia, for instance, or that dreaded trip to the ICU).

Two days after my mother was admitted to the community hospital, a local orthopedic surgeon, someone we met only an hour before the surgery, performed a hemiarthroplasty (partial hip replacement), inserting a prosthetic femoral head into my mother's hip socket and anchoring the stem of that head in her femur bone. It was a quick and fairly straightforward procedure.

"She has pretty good bone structure for her age," the surgeon told us as we sat in the waiting room after the surgery. "The operation was a success."

Of course it was. That's my mom, bulling her way through another adverse situation.

But our own education was just beginning. Even as someone who knows health care quite well, I felt like an uneducated fool in this instance. What I found out as soon as my mother got back to her room the evening of the surgery is that with joint replacements now, you are on a quick-moving assembly line. That line whips you out of the hospital and into a rehab facility as fast as is humanly possible, and then out of the rehab facility and either home or to a nursing home almost as quickly.

My mother was now participating in a pilot program created by the Centers for Medicare and Medicaid Services (CMS) in 2016, part of the agency's broader "bundled payment" initiative. This particular pilot program placed hospitals at financial risk for joint replacements if the total costs of care from the surgery through a certain number of days after being discharged from the hospital exceeded a certain amount. The program did this through a form of payment bundling, in which Medicare added up the actual total costs of care for a patient getting a joint replacement over a period of time (called "the care episode") and compared it to a "target price" it set, which was what CMS estimated the total costs should be. Spending more than the CMS target price across the entire continuum of care for a hip replacement, including rehabilitation, could force the hospital to reimburse Medicare for a portion of the total costs, while coming in under the target price might give the hospital a financial bonus.

The problem was that no one told us before the surgery, or for several days afterward, that my mother was going to be a participant in this program. I found out only after a chance mention by the hospital "care manager" when she was discussing my mother's discharge with me over the phone on the day my mother was scheduled to be moved to the rehab facility. I think if I had not peppered her with highly specific questions about length-of-stay and expected Medicare Part A coverage for rehabilitation, she might have never mentioned the bundled payment program. My brother also had spoken with this care manager several times before, but my mother's inclusion in the program had never come up. It was as if the care manager shared the information only on a "need-to-know" basis, though this was something I felt sure we all needed to know, even before the surgery.

Learning about Bundles

The first 24 hours after surgery were a flurry of activity. My brother and sister remained with our mom in the hospital while I went back home to attend to other family obligations. The morning after her surgery, my mother was forced out of her bed to sit in a chair and to try and stand. She yelled at staff members the whole time, her dementia on full display. Sure, it sounds like it makes sense clinically: Get them up quick and get them moving. But the speed with which things started happening struck my siblings and me as less than ideal. It also made me wonder, looking back, if there wasn't some conflict of interest on the hospital's part—regardless of the clinical appropriateness of what happened to my mother—given her membership in this new bundled payment program, which seems to encourage hospitals to move joint replacement patients quickly to somewhere else.

The day before the surgery, we had been told that my mother would be discharged no more than a couple of days later to a rehabilitation facility. Given the short discharge window, my brother and I had spent the morning of the surgery, a Friday, doing a lightning tour of a local rehab hospital that we'd selected after my own rapid-fire examination of Medicare Star Ratings, Nursing Home Compare data, and New York State Department of Health inspection reports. Thankfully I knew something about health care quality measures; for other people, this process might take a lot longer. The care manager needed to know the name of the facility we wanted my mother discharged to because she would be brought there on the Monday following surgery. Over that weekend, I remained baffled by how fast the situation was moving, and I dreaded the coming week.

The hospital had recommended one specific rehabilitation hospital, but once I did my own research, another local facility seemed to offer the best quality. Later, when I learned that the hospital was at risk financially for the total costs of the continuum of my mother's care, the idea of a conflict of interest again filled my head. Was there something about my mother's inclusion in the payment bundle that had made the hospital recommend or do things that were not in her best interest? More specifically, did the hospital have tacit understandings with specific rehab facilities about the need to keep the overall costs of care within a certain range? Was the hospital's recommendation reflective of good collaboration or something more like collusion with a given facility? I can't say whether my suspicions had much basis in reality. But my trust in that hospital and my mother's surgeon began to wane.

The day of the discharge, after my phone call with the care manager, I tried to read up on the bundled payment program. Online I found an item from the *Federal Register* that was more than 280 pages long and 48 pages of "frequently asked questions" describing the program to health care providers. For patients and families, I found an oversimplified set of statements on the CMS website, including many still unproven assertions that bundled payment produces better care for patients. All of the information I found made my head hurt. It felt as if my mother's care trajectory had been reduced to thousands of hard-to-understand words online.

I was confused and angry. I tried not to laugh out loud at the grand-sounding but vague statements about "coordinated patient-centered care," the benefits of hospitals and providers "working together more closely to coordinate their care," and how bundling created incentives to "work together to deliver more effective and efficient care."

I know enough about health care to understand that these sentiments often do not translate well in the siloed, hypercompetitive, slim-profit-margin system of care delivery that we have today.

What my siblings and I saw during the first week my mother was in the rehabilitation facility made me feel as if the "bundle" in which she had been captured was working against and not for her. A 90-year-old with dementia, my mother is a unique patient with special circumstances. Yet my siblings and I were told initially that, on average, participation in the bundled program meant five days of Medicare Part A–covered rehabilitation for a partial hip replacement.

Every time I spoke with the rehabilitation facility staff members in that first week, I could feel that this bundled payment program and its short discharge window were on their minds.

"You know your mother is part of a care bundle," a nurse on my mother's floor mentioned to me one day.

In separate instances, the physical therapist and the social worker in charge of my mom's health care team mentioned that to me as well.

I also found out that the rehabilitation facility was in constant communication with the care manager at the hospital that had discharged my mother, providing regular progress reports. This might have been to help coordinate my mother's postsurgical care and ensure that it was successful. In fact, I didn't doubt that. But the cynic in me also wondered how the rehabilitation facility would get future referrals from the hospital without being able to show the hospital that the facility could make the bundle a financial success through highly efficient service delivery. There was little transparency about the relationship between the institutions for my siblings and me. And right or wrong, my trust in the rehabilitation facility began to erode as well.

A little more than a week into my mom's stay in the rehab facility, after it had become clear that she could not be discharged in five days because of her slow response to physical therapy, we had a family meeting with my mother's health care team. I joined in by phone from Boston. The team members told us that the facility was close to reporting to the hospital and Medicare that they had reached the limit of rehabilitation progress with my mother, which would trigger her transition to a "private pay" patient and end the rehab facility's obligation under the joint replacement bundle. This would likely also make the hospital happier and end its obligation, I thought.

My mother wasn't progressing, the team members said. At times, she refused to cooperate in her rehabilitation, and the facility needed to report to the hospital and Medicare when progress was slowing.

The meeting got heated in a hurry. I countered the team's standardized responses with my own questions.

"You have to realize my mother has dementia and has to be treated differently—are you taking that into account?" I asked.

My brother joined in as well from the conference room. We pressed the team on the fact that my mother's dementia and other secondary morbidities she was dealing with, such as chronic knee pain, were likely slowing down her physical therapy progress compared to that of a "typical patient."

"I can't believe we have to state what should be obvious," I said.

Again and again, I brought up the pressures of the dreaded bundle program. I wanted everyone in the room to know that we knew about it. It seemed a subtle (maybe not so subtle, in hindsight) form of shaming that might get them to think like advocates for my mother. For 45 minutes, this back-and-forth continued between the dry, clinical analysis from the care team and the emotional, frustrated pleas from my brother and me. This was nothing like what the CMS website talked about. After the call, I left my office, feeling sick to my stomach, and went outside to clear my head. I felt increasingly powerless to help my mother.

An Unrealistic Policy

For years I've believed and taught my students that fee-for-service medicine was a wasteful, dysfunctional way to reimburse providers for health care. Maybe it still is. But I now think that value-based reimbursement, the supposed antidote, often makes little sense and is equally dysfunctional, at least from the patient's perspective. It can create a massive conflict of interest within a system that is neither coordinated nor collaborative, and whose institutions are still very much concerned first and foremost with profit. Bundled payment? Well, that makes even less sense to me now. I don't see how there won't be conflict, tension, and ultimately gaming going on between hospitals and the downstream facilities that care for their patients.

Ironically, my mother is still in that same facility, now situated in a long-term-care bed that Medicare is not paying for. Her staying put is less by choice and more by necessity, since the facility is close to where my brother and sister live, so they can see her every day. In addition, it was the only place we considered that had a long-term-care bed available. In the end, the facility kept her on Medicare Part A coverage for five weeks because of some meaningful setbacks to her rehabilitation that, to anyone's eye, justified keeping her for even longer—and, I think, because we had pushed back hard in that meeting. The handful of days in rehab that we were told was typical for hip replacements within the bundled payment program was, at least in my mother's case, a ridiculously unrealistic length of time. Even five weeks of rehab seemed insufficient: at the end of it, she was still not back to her previous level of functioning, and to this day she hardly ever gets out of her wheelchair. I credit the rehabilitation facility for justifying to both the hospital and Medicare a need to cover her care longer. But I wonder if they have learned a hard lesson that they will apply in less patient-friendly ways in the future as value-based payment experiments continue.

I know that if my mother could understand the reimbursement world in which she had been dropped, she would fume. Her fiery temper would have given the providers around her no quarter, and in the end many of them would've known firsthand what this new reimbursement system means to the patient. Instead, my brother and I have tried to channel her response. I write this story because she would expect me to. After all, she raised us to rail against things that seem unfair or downright hostile. I certainly don't think that value-based reimbursement, especially through what are called "comprehensive payment bundles for specific care episodes," is fair to the patient. These bundles may sound great on paper but not from my perspective. Instead of paying full attention to my mother and her feelings, my siblings and I had to be hypervigilant agitators within the health care system—a system that listened to us best when we took an adversarial posture. This is not the fulfillment of the patient-centered care goal that CMS so desires. It's far from it.

That is the lesson I will teach now to my students and anyone else who will listen.

Even in an Emergency, Doctors Must Make Informed Consent an Informed Choice

When a stroke is suspected, a daughter is pressured to consent to her father's treatment without fully understanding the risks.

Cindy Brach

My dad is a wonderful man. In his working years, he was a tax accountant who served on the board of the Bronx River Neighborhood Center and shared his passion for tennis by teaching young men who lived in the South Bronx to play. He retired early to introduce others to meditation and other stress reduction methods that he had found helpful, and he ended up as a volunteer community mediator.

In October 2013, just a few months after giving up playing tennis, my 88-year-old father was diagnosed as having stage IV prostate cancer. He responded well to the hormone treatments, but by May 2014 his prostate had gotten so large that he had difficulty peeing. Although he liked saying, "I don't like to brag, but I have a HUUUGE prostate," this condition had become dangerous: the blockage began to cause kidney failure.

My dad's urologist gave him two choices. He could either live with a catheter (a tube inserted into his bladder) for the rest of his life, or he could have surgery to trim his prostate to create a channel for the pee. After hearing that sporting a catheter would end his Ping-Pong career and that he'd only have to spend one night in the hospital, my dad overcame a long-standing fear of germs and elected to have the surgery.

Volume 35, Number 4. April 2016.
Editor's Note: The views expressed in this article are those of the author, who is responsible for its content, and do not necessarily represent the views of the Agency for Healthcare Research and Quality (AHRQ). No statement in this article should be construed as an official position of AHRQ or of the US Department of Health and Human Services.

Since my mother's immune system was shot from having chemo-therapy for lymphoma, my 20-year-old son and I were the ones who accompanied my dad to the hospital. I am not a clinician, but I have worked for the Agency for Healthcare Research and Quality for al-most 20 years, and I felt well equipped to be my dad's health care proxy. He checked into the ambulatory surgery unit early in the morning and was soon taken away for the surgery.

Complications after Surgery

Immediately after the surgery, my dad's urologist told us that it had gone well. The following morning, however, he informed us there was too much blood in my dad's pee. My father had to stay in the hospital an extra day so they could flush the blood out while the cath-eter was still in place.

On his third day in the hospital, my father was pronounced ready for a "voiding trial." They pumped a liter of fluid into his bladder, removed the catheter, and waited to see if he could pee. However, my dad felt no urge to go. Even after drinking cup after cup of water and sitting with a handheld urinal for several hours, he couldn't get anything out.

It was early that afternoon when I noticed that he was having some difficulty speaking. He was clearly trying to say something but couldn't come up with the words he was searching for.

I pointed out the problem to the urology nurse practitioner.

"Dad, what are you trying to do?" I asked him.

"Well, I'm trying to . . ." His words trailed off. "You see, I'm mak-ing an effort . . . I'm really . . ." He couldn't say, "I'm trying to pee."

The nurse practitioner suggested that we call the stroke team. While I didn't think my dad had had a stroke, I knew I might be at-tributing the symptoms to other health issues, which frequently hap-pens to stroke victims in hospitals. So I agreed, and the nurse called in the stroke team.

Strong-Arm Tactics

Fifteen minutes later half a dozen neurology residents were swarming around the room. One of them performed the standard stroke assessment—how many fingers do you see, squeeze my fingers, hold your arms out and don't let me push them down, and so on.

The next thing I knew, they were rolling my dad out the door on a gurney.

"Where are you taking him?" I asked.

"To the ER to give him tPA," the lead resident answered as they wheeled him down the hall. I knew what tPA was: tissue plasminogen activator, a stroke treatment drug that busts up clots that block the flow of blood to the brain. But I was not convinced that my dad was having a stroke.

"But I haven't consented," I called after them.

"This is an emergency!" they replied.

I stood my ground. "I'm his health proxy. You're NOT giving him anything without my consent, and I haven't consented!" That stopped them.

"You're right," the resident said, backpedaling. "Could you come with us while I explain?"

As I trotted to the elevator with them, the resident explained that my father had had a stroke, that there was medicine they could give to break up the blood clot, but that there was a short window of time in which the medicine could be administered.

How could they be so sure he'd had a stroke? I wondered to myself. Did they know my dad had been too shaky on his feet to take a walk that morning, that he had not eaten until the nurse made him have a yogurt midmorning, and that he later threw up his lunch? Did they know that he hadn't slept much the past two nights? Could it be that his full bladder was causing his kidneys to go toxic again?

I'd seen my dad get fuzzy when he had a bladder infection—maybe that was the problem. Or maybe the exhaustion from trying to pass the "voiding trial" and the worry about the pain he'd feel if they had to put the catheter back in were affecting my elderly father.

Maybe I'd watched too many episodes of the medical drama *House*, but it seemed as if the doctors hadn't ruled out other possible causes of my dad's symptom. They hadn't asked me anything about his history other than the time of the onset of symptoms. I was worried that these neurologists in training might see a stroke where there wasn't one because that's what they were looking for.

"Why are you so sure it's a stroke?" I asked the lead resident. "Was there anything other than the language problem?"

No, the resident answered, there was nothing else.

On the way to the emergency department (ED), we stopped for my father to get a CT scan to make sure he wasn't already bleeding into his brain, which is a contraindication for administering tPA. All I had heard thus far was how tPA could reverse stroke symptoms—no one had told me about any potential downsides. I asked the stroke team about the risks from tPA if my father was not having a stroke. I was told there was a small risk (on the order of 1 percent) that tPA would cause him to bleed into his brain, which could either kill him or leave him severely impaired. No one bothered to mention that the risk of a catastrophic brain bleed from tPA was even greater if he was in fact having a stroke. Or that there was a risk of a noncatastrophic brain bleed.

The CT scan showed no bleeding. As we moved quickly on to the ED, I was pressed for my consent to give my father tPA.

"It's the standard of care!" the resident kept hammering at me. "We're running out of time."

I repeated that I had not consented and proceeded to call my mother. She and I were both my father's health care proxies. While I was on the phone explaining the situation to my mother, a senior neurology resident interrupted me to make sure I *really* understood that time was running out. I put my mom on speakerphone so she could hear what the senior resident had to say, which was what I'd already been told: that tPA would break up the clot, that tPA was the standard of care, and that it was critical for my father to get the medicine right away.

I took my mother off speakerphone so we could discuss the decision, but the senior resident insisted that I give her a decision right then. I gave her the response I'd often given my children when they pestered me for an immediate answer, "If you need an answer now, the answer is no."

On the phone, my mother gave her opinion. Maybe it was just that tPA had received good press coverage, she said, but she wanted my dad to get the medicine. So I consented. It was barely within the three-hour treatment window when they administered the drug.

Shortly after receiving the drug, as my dad was being wheeled up to the neurology unit, he sat halfway up with outstretched arms, shook violently, and then lay back down. "He's having a seizure," someone cried, at which point he seized a second time.

My father had suffered from an intracranial hemorrhage—he had bled into his brain. Throughout the rest of that night in the neurology intensive care unit, he shook uncontrollably, didn't appear to understand us, and couldn't communicate at all. Tears streamed down my face.

What had I done? Had my mistake been to allow them to give him the tPA? Or had it been in questioning its administration in the first place and losing valuable time? Why, despite being an expert on health literacy who was developing training modules to improve informed consent in hospitals, was I unable to come up with the questions to get the information I needed to make a truly informed choice in a timely manner?

My dad trusted me to make good decisions for him, and I felt I had let him down. I also felt the hospital staff had let me down.

Health care systems can and must do a better job. What would have served me and my family during my father's emergency was better communication and a care team geared to helping us reach a treatment decision.

Improving Communication

Clinical trials have shown, on average, more benefit than harm for the average patient meeting specified stroke criteria when tPA is administered within three to four hours of the first symptoms. The earlier the patient receives the medicine, the better the results. This creates both intense time pressure and the illusion that there is no time to spare for conversations. But if clinicians can communicate effectively and efficiently, the time can be found.

Doctors are the experts in medicine. Patients and their families are the experts in themselves and their bodies. The neurology residents who evaluated my father for stroke should also have been asking me questions. They should have asked about what my father was normally like, whether he had ever experienced symptoms like this before, if I knew of anything that might account for his current symptom, and other questions to gather more evidence about his condition.

Had the residents taken more seriously my doubts about whether my dad had had a stroke and my concerns about the treatment, they might have told me that they had checked my father's blood sugar level, and that there was a second symptom of stroke they hadn't told me about. Instead, valuable time was wasted, and I was left confused and in turmoil.

There is a growing expectation that doctors should be effective communicators. Medical schools have begun to teach communication skills, especially since the United States Medical Licensing Examination started testing those skills with the use of simulated patients in 2004, and the communication skills component of the exam was enhanced in 2012. Additionally, the results of surveys of patients' experiences of care—which include questions about how well doctors and nurses respect, listen to, and explain things clearly to patients—are being used in determining hospital payments. But we still have a long way to go. Hospital leaders need to make it known throughout their organization that clear communication is an institutional priority.

Every discussion of possible treatments should cover the risks, harms, and benefits of all the options—including the option of doing nothing. This is a basic tenet of informed consent, which unfortunately many hospitals do not observe. Hospitals have been cited by the Joint Commission for failing to have appropriate informed consent policies in place, but little attention has been paid to whether they adhere to the policies they have established.

In my dad's case, the residents should have educated me about the natural progression of stroke and the chances that the stroke would resolve on its own, that the symptoms would persist or increase, or that the stroke would kill him. They should have taken me through a similar risk-benefit discussion of tPA and explained the chances that my father would improve, stay the same, get worse, or die.

Risk communication is notoriously difficult. One method used to simplify the task is a visual representation of the risks and benefits of a treatment versus other alternatives. Since my father's emergency, I've considered whether something like this would have helped me.

One challenge is making such illustrations unbiased. My research found two graphics showing the benefits and risks of tPA, but both were criticized by Jigneshkumar Gadhia and colleagues in a review article published in 2010 in *Stroke* for presenting a distorted view of the risks and benefits. Furthermore, these types of graphics are complex and can be difficult to understand, even for patients with high health literacy, as noted by Jasmir Nayak and colleagues in a 2015 article in *Patient Education and Counseling*.

Another problem is that the graphics show the aggregate results of clinical trials. For graphics to be meaningful communication tools, they need to depict the risks and benefits for each patient as accurately as possible. Some work has been done to tailor risk-benefit calculations to patients using data from stroke registries and to present these data to patients and families. This would not only have given the residents treating my dad more precise guidance, but it would also have allayed my concerns that the treatment they recommended was dictated by a rule of thumb instead of my father's particular situation.

Translating the results into easy-to-understand graphics remains challenging, however. Testing these tools with diverse patients, including those with limited health literacy, will be essential.

Making Informed Consent an Informed Choice

Some people would argue that stroke treatment is not an area that should be subject to shared decision-making. They would say that the science is clear and that a doctor's objective should be to obtain consent as quickly as possible to increase the likelihood of a good outcome. Some patients and family members would indeed prefer to abdicate the decision to clinicians. That is their prerogative. I believe that patients and family members have a role to play, even when decisions must be made quickly. The claim that "it's an emergency" does not exempt clinicians from engaging patients and families and explaining the situation in an understandable way so that if consent is given, it is truly informed. Evidence should never be used as a cudgel to pressure patients to consent to treatments they don't fully understand.

Different people will be prepared to take different risks. Some people will feel better if they avail themselves of a chance for a full recovery, even if the treatment involved is risky. Others will feel worse if they gave their consent for something that ended up killing their loved one. There will always be bad outcomes, and how patients and their families feel when they occur matters. After all, patients and families have to live with the consequences.

The informed consent process has to be more than chasing down a signature for a form. To empower patients and families to make informed choices, health care organizations must build supportive systems. For example, hospitals could maintain a library of high-quality decision aids, which are tools designed to facilitate shared decision-making and patient participation in health care decisions. Even the most dedicated doctors will have difficulty engaging patients and families in shared decision-making without the support of their institutions.

Making Engagement Part of the Protocol

Hospitals' "door-to-needle time"—the time between when a stroke patient arrives and when tPA is administered—is now a quality metric. There has been a major push to increase the number of stroke patients who receive the drug quickly. Protocol dictates that when a stroke is suspected in the hospital, a stroke team is called to evaluate the patient. If the patient meets the criteria for tPA, a CT scan is done, and if there are no signs of a brain bleed, tPA is administered.

To turn informed consent into informed choice, patient and family engagement has to be integrated into this protocol. It could dictate, for example, that while the patient is being evaluated, a member of the stroke team lets family members know that a decision may have to be made quickly and asks if any other relatives should be involved in the decision.

The protocol could also specify that during the CT scan, the family be briefed about the results of the evaluation, the purpose of the scan, and the upcoming decision about whether to administer tPA. The next step would call for the doctor to sit down with the patient and family and use a personalized decision aid to elicit their goals and preferences. After discussing the benefits, harms, and risks of the options, including the option of no treatment, the doctor would check that this information had been understood. The final step would be that the doctor helps the patient and family make a choice. Everything could be accomplished in a short amount of time if the process was streamlined and clearly delineated.

Simply having a policy in place that doctors must obtain informed consent is not sufficient. To make sure that patients and families are appropriately included in decision-making every time, roles need to be specified (for example, who is going to explain the results of the stroke assessment), logistics need to be worked out (for instance, where there is a place to talk, or how family members who are not on site will be contacted if cell phones don't work in the ED), and staff members have to be trained (for example, how to use decision aids, engage patients and families in the decision-making process, and check their understanding of the information they've been given).

In addition, adherence to policies about patient and family inclusion has to be monitored. And when policies are not followed, these failures should be studied to determine where the breakdown occurred and what corrective action is needed.

Epilogue

My father was lucky. He got back most of his functioning after the brain bleed, although he can only play Ping-Pong sitting down and can no longer go out for a walk by himself because he is at risk of falling or getting disoriented. The doctors are pleased with the outcome, but I am displeased that they did not explain the risks before I gave consent. The health care system needs to hardwire patient and family engagement into the informed consent process, even in emergencies.

When the residents gave my father a stroke diagnosis, I needed someone to serve as an unbiased interpreter of the evidence, to recognize my knowledge of this particular patient, and to ask about our values and goals. I needed someone to acknowledge that we faced a hard decision, that there were no guarantees, and that it was ultimately our choice. Anything less violates the principles of informed consent and the dignity of patients and families.

4

The Doctor-Patient Relationship

How to Win the Doctor Lottery

Not every doctor-patient encounter is healing, and it can seem a game of chance. One patient explores what it takes to win.

Donna Jackson Nakazawa

When my son was five weeks old, he began to turn away from my breast even when hungry. He'd suck, then cry sharply, and twist away. I called the office of the pediatrician I'd chosen while pregnant, but she had no free appointments, so I saw another doctor in the practice instead. I'll call him Dr. Jones. He examined my son, told me he had "gas pains," and asked me, "Are you feeling anxious about being a good mom?"

The next day my son seemed better. *Was* I overly anxious, I asked myself? Then my son projectile vomited across the bedroom. I strapped him in his car seat and headed back to the doctor. Dr. Jones asked his nurse to take me aside for a "mom heart-to-heart." Being a new mom is anxiety-inducing, the nurse said, adding, "What are you doing for you?" I burst into tears. They must have thought I was a postpartum hormonal time bomb.

The next morning when my son tried to breastfeed, he stopped and screamed in a way that resonated within my cells. That cell-shock sensation was something I'd felt only once before in my life.

Three decades earlier, at the age of 12, I'd stood at the side of my father's hospital bed after he'd undergone a bowel resection, a "routine" gastrointestinal surgery. Every grown-up had told me that my dad would be fine despite postoperative complications. But as I looked into my father's eyes that afternoon, I saw a depth of pain-laced love and the anticipation of loss reflected there. My earth tipped on its axis. I suddenly knew that despite what everyone was telling me, my father would not be fine.

That night, at the age of 42, my father died.

Racing to Save My Child

I arrived at the pediatrician's office on the third morning of my son's unexplained distress. As I began to explain why I was there, Dr. Jones interrupted me, gave me a handout on colic and a pat on the back, and ushered me out.

Just at that moment, my son's original doctor—the one I'd joined the practice to see—stepped out of another room and saw me standing in the hallway.

"Haven't I seen you here every day?" she asked. Her eyes were kind. I nodded, swallowing back tears.

"Let's see your baby." She extended her arms and laid my son on the exam table, gently palpating his abdomen. "Tell me about when you first felt something wasn't right? What else have you been noticing?"

She took a bottle of breast milk from my hands and offered it to my son. He sucked, turned beet red, and twisted away with a sob. "Does he do this on the breast, too?"

I nodded.

Then she uttered the words that would save my son's life. "I listen to my moms," she said. "Given what I'm observing, I'd like to get an abdominal sonogram."

"But they told me it's colic." I suddenly hoped Dr. Jones had been right.

"His abdomen seems distended and hard," she said. "It's a subtle finding, but it's there."

A few hours later, after the sonogram, the pediatrician held the hospital's report. It suggested pyloric stenosis, a condition caused by a tight muscle that prevents food from exiting the stomach and entering the intestines. When that muscle becomes rigid, it resembles an olive.

"I don't find this definitive," she continued. "I've called a pediatric surgeon at Hopkins. He'll meet you at the ER. Pack what you'll need for the next week."

I held my son, his tired exhales warm and moist against my neck. "Johns Hopkins?" I asked. That was where my father had died.

She put her hand on my arm. "I know this is difficult. But I promise you, we will help your baby. We will get through this."

She handed me a slip of paper. "Here's my cell. Call when you've arrived."

I held the paper like a talisman.

Later that afternoon, the Hopkins surgeon examined my son, rubbing his thumb over his belly, looking for the swollen muscle the local hospital said they'd seen. "Pyloric stenosis my eye!" he nearly roared. "There's no olive here!"

The new tests he wanted to run seemed invasive, and our pediatrician called to reassure my husband and me. "Please, trust us with your baby," she said. "This is a cautious, but necessary, path."

That evening, we stood outside of a glass-walled room while our son underwent a barium drop X-ray of his gastrointestinal tract. Suddenly, the radiologist screamed. She picked up the phone and called the surgeon. "You have to see this! His intestines are wrapped north of his stomach! They're about to twist off!" The surgeon arrived and operated on our son, unfurling his intestines, removing 21 adhesions, and carefully placing his bowels back in.

Weeks later, after we brought our son home, his recovery was tenuous. Some days, we ended up back at the hospital. Our surgeon called for nightly reports on bowel sounds. Once, we met our pediatrician at her office at eleven o'clock at night; another time, she examined our son's abdomen on a bench at her son's athletic game to ensure that his postoperative discomfort was nonsurgical. Each time we saw each other during that year—and often in the two decades since—we hugged, blinking back tears. As my son began to live a normal boy's life, we sighed relief. He was, we agreed, "the one who almost got away."

Winning, or Losing, the Doctor Lottery

Today, my son is six foot two and a senior in college. When he was a newborn, his three-inch scar extended across his belly. Today that scar appears deceivingly small. In the decades since, his case has been taught in medical schools and used in lawsuits by parents whose pediatricians hadn't listened and whose children had needlessly died.

Why were we so fortunate? I didn't know it two decades ago, but despite the terror of those weeks in which we almost lost our child, something good, and rare, had happened. We had won what I've since come to call the "Doctor Lottery."

When you win the Doctor Lottery, there is no cash prize but a far greater payoff: the possibility of extraordinary healing, even a miracle. Our son survived because our physician took the time to listen, show compassion, earn trust, partner with us, advocate, and provide just the right amount of care to save a life. She fostered a safe and healing patient-doctor relationship while navigating us through a sea of uncertainty.

My family and I haven't always won the Doctor Lottery. My father's surgeon, for instance, had pushed him to have the bowel resection to "cure" him of diverticulitis, a disease in which the colon's lining becomes inflamed. He stitched up my father's intestines with a suture known to dissolve in patients who've been on steroids and hadn't read my father's chart to see that his internist had recently had him on cortisone. Nor did he look at the list of medications my father had carefully written down on his patient intake forms. When the sutures dissolved, my father, who had a bleeding disorder, went into shock. His abdomen was distended and hard.

My mother asked the nurse to page the surgeon. "My husband is in so much pain!" she said. The surgeon, who was playing golf, told the nurse to tell my mother, "Pain after surgery is normal." By the time my father developed a fever, and peritonitis, it was too late. He died of a heart attack. "Normal courses of antibiotics proved unsuccessful," my father's death report reads.

Not only did we not win the Doctor Lottery that day, but my brothers and I lost our childhood. When my father passed away, the world as we knew it ended, as if someone had erased all the color from the horizon.

My Turn in the Lottery

These experiences informed my own health journey when, in 2001, I became a revolving-door hospital patient facing two long periods of paralysis from Guillain-Barré syndrome, a neurological autoimmune disease similar to multiple sclerosis. The day my Hopkins neurologist delivered the diagnosis, I passed through a portal into a terrifying and unknown universe.

As my husband filled out admission papers, my neurologist sat beside my wheelchair, quietly explaining the treatment I would undergo. He would start infusions of other people's healthy immune cells to try to reverse my paralysis. After he finished talking, we sat together in silence. Nurses rapped at the door. His patient waiting room filled. But he never left my side. I asked him why he stayed with me when he had so much to do—he was, after all, the head of a major department. He told me, his eyes looking into mine, "I will not leave you sitting here alone, not with the news I've just given you."

Over the next few months, I slowly learned to walk again. But, although Guillain-Barré syndrome rarely strikes the same patient twice, four years later I developed it again. This time, I fell into a state of paralysis faster, and the damage to my nerves was more extensive. During my hospitalization, several of my doctor's fellow neurologists warned me to "hope for the best but prepare for the worst." They said that I might never get out of a wheelchair. But my neurologist shook his head and reassured me that some people did recover. He thought I could, too. "Don't listen to them," he told me. "I'm your doctor, I know you."

His words stayed with me during that hot slog of summer into fall, as I sweated in rehab, then through grueling physical therapy at home that left me shuddering and depleted.

Eventually, six months later, I was able to navigate steps with a cane and then walk out my front door and down the driveway.

Finding a Physician-Partner

Some months later, however, like many Guillain-Barré syndrome patients, I still navigated through a flu-like fatigue. I'd also developed symptoms of gastroparesis, a condition in which the stomach can't empty itself normally. A new, local doctor I saw seemed to think me a hysteric and handed me Prilosec. I will never forget the look of disdain on his face the second time I saw him, and he said, "A few days ago you came in saying you were nauseated, and today you say you have diarrhea! Make up your mind!"

I sought out a number of physicians, seeking answers, until in 2011 I met a new internist, Anastasia Rowland-Seymour, at Johns Hopkins, who changed my life by partnering with me to create a new health story.

Dr. Rowland-Seymour asked me gently about my history, never looking at her computer. I told her that I knew I was lucky to be doing so well, walking, driving. I told her of my bone-deep fatigue, numbness, headaches, and that I often found myself so tired I had to lie down on the floor after climbing the stairs. "That's my normal," I said with a shrug. I figured our time was up, but she wanted to have a deeper conversation about my well-being.

"You've been through a great deal in a relatively short period of time." She looked as if she didn't quite buy my breezy rendition. "That has to have taken quite a toll on you."

She wondered if I thought that the decades of stress I'd endured might have played a role in the immune dysfunction I now faced. She asked me if my childhood, in particular, had been stressful.

I was astonished.

"I've never thought about it that way," I said, telling her, in briefest terms, about my father's sudden death.

That day, I found a partner on my path to healing, one who helped me incrementally incorporate mind-body approaches to well-being with conventional medical care. Over the next year, my health dramatically improved.

After having seen the best and worst of medicine over three generations, I've learned that people suffer needlessly, or pursue new possibilities of healing, based largely on whether they have a healing doctor-patient partnership.

I've seen this pattern in my work as a science journalist, too. I've heard from thousands of patients about relationships with doctors that helped—or hindered—their health and recovery. It's clear that the tenor and quality of the patient-doctor relationship play a telling role.

Every patient wants and deserves to win the Doctor Lottery; it shouldn't be simply a matter of chance. The good news is that I believe we can get there, in three key ways.

Feeling Known

In my healing encounters with physicians, I felt that I was being heard, understood, and respected. My internist, Dr. Rowland-Seymour, now at the Case Western Reserve School of Medicine, trains medical students in gaining skills to create a sense of safety and partnership with their patients. Through simulated role-playing exercises, she shows students how to create trust from the moment they meet a patient, such as by letting the patient walk in the room and sit down first and asking open-ended questions such as, "What else is coming up for you?"

A 2015 study in *Narrative Inquiry in Bioethics* found that patients overwhelmingly felt that what mattered most was having a physician who listened, acknowledged their condition, was honest, and treated them as an equal. A 2006 study in the *Journal of General Internal Medicine* found that the single greatest predictor of whether patients with HIV adhered to treatment was whether they felt "known as a person" by their physician.

The first time I met Dr. Rowland-Seymour, I entered the exam room ready to focus on managing symptoms. I was surprised to discover that past trauma might also need to be addressed if I hoped to improve.

When physicians don't take the time to listen and be present, their patients are less likely to trust their decisions. In a 2015 study in *JAMA Oncology*, patients with poor relationships with their physicians were more likely to demand added tests and procedures.

"We know that when people feel they have been fully heard and seen in a relationship, they are more likely to heal," says Bob Whitaker, a professor of public health and pediatrics at Temple University. That's helpful to a patient even before doctors intervene with traditional medicine, he adds.

When I think of the extraordinary doctors in my family's healing stories, they shared something in common. They were deeply present during our encounters, as if they were there to stand shoulder to shoulder with us—rather than simply to give directives. Because they established that rapport, they helped us navigate uncertainty in the face of terror while still championing real hope for recovery.

This doesn't mean offering a patient false hope, Dr. Rowland-Seymour underscores, but rather "a sense that we are going to figure out how to manage this, and get you better, and we are going to do it as a team."

Understanding Past Trauma

Most physicians are trained to "walk around trauma as the elephant in the room," Dr. Rowland-Seymour says. If they don't see a direct correlation between how trauma has affected a patient's well-being and long-term health, they sidestep it. But you can't achieve true healing with that elephant in the room.

Jeffrey Brenner, a 2013 MacArthur "Genius" Fellow and senior vice president of integrated health and human services at UnitedHealthcare, where he leads myConnections, a program to pilot new models of health care, is an advocate for training medical students to screen patients for trauma. He has found in his own clinic that knowing about patients' early-life trauma "is as important as knowing their vital signs."

When physicians grasp that past trauma can affect current physical health, they can also better understand why poor health habits might be coping mechanisms for past wounds, and why it is especially difficult for some patients to engage in the kind of self-care that's critical to healing.

Trauma awareness also helps physicians recognize their own past trauma and stress. According to Henry Weil of the Columbia University College of Physicians and Surgeons, the physician who has developed self-awareness of his or her own suffering, and the effect that trauma has had on his or her life, is often best able to view patient suffering "with an open heart."

Realigning Incentives

Even when new doctors are trained to foster a strong patient-doctor relationship and recognize trauma, the system all too often pushes them in the opposite direction. After medical school, physicians quickly learn that they're better rewarded for moving fast than for taking a thorough patient history. In a hospital clinic setting, internists have 15 minutes to see each patient, which might be fine if the patient has a sore throat, but in large teaching hospitals, most patients are struggling with multiple, complex chronic conditions.

The physicians with whom I've spoken agree that doctors who put in the extra time to create relationships with patients do it because they feel it is the right thing to do, despite the fact that the system doesn't reward their efforts. But a system that relies on physician good-heartedness alone is hardly sustainable, especially given that half of physicians already report professional burnout.

The good news is that a quiet revolution is now afoot in medicine. Many doctors, just like their patients, long to have more healing encounters and foster strong patient-doctor relationships. To achieve that, we will have to rethink how we deliver medicine.

How to Shift the Paradigm

Ensuring that more doctors know how to foster a healing relationship means that medical schools will need to reenvision how they select the right students and deepen their training. This goes beyond teaching students and interns to maintain eye contact or use open-ended inquiry. It will require teaching mindful, empathic listening and rewarding doctors-in-training for developing strong patient-doctor communication skills and relationships. Compassion and empathy training—tailored to the physician experience—are particularly important during the grueling years of medical training, but all doctors should revisit these skills as part of continued medical education.

We also need to revisit how time during the face-to-face patient encounter is being used.

"Good things have come from technology, but technology can't do everything we thought it could," Dr. Whitaker, of Temple University, says. "If a physician has their back to the patient, and is looking at the computer while taking a patient history, that's not a healing encounter."

As Dr. Rowland-Seymour pointed out to me, dentists often have a scribe taking notes while they do a dental exam, but internists don't. Trying to connect with patients while staring at a computer screen just doesn't make sense. Vikas Saini, president of the Lown Institute, suggests incentivizing the development of systems that use voice recognition software and artificial intelligence to extract relevant patient data from voice or video recordings, thus freeing the physician to be more present with patients.

Primary care physicians and other providers are already helping drive the types of changes that make it more likely patients will win the Doctor Lottery. For one, they are moving toward value-based care delivery and payment models, which reward meeting quality-of-care targets as opposed to simply paying for the quantity of care. Team-based care, in which a doctor works as a member of a larger team (including, for instance, a medical assistant, social worker, and behavioral health expert), also can create a more healing environment and ensure that all of a patient's needs are addressed. Lastly, greater attention is being paid to transitions in care, to ensure that care runs smoothly across various settings, especially when multiple providers are involved, so that life-saving information is never lost in translation. All of these strategies rely upon doctors listening to, seeing, and respecting their patients—and on measuring care not only by their actions but by their presence.

But real change won't happen unless physicians place value on these qualities within themselves and within the profession.

I only wish it weren't too late for my father to have won the Doctor Lottery. His unnecessary death inspired me to insist on having doctors who listened and treated me with respect. It is bittersweet that my dad's unintentional legacy was the very gift that would help me reclaim my health and save the life of the grandson who, sadly, he never got to meet.

At the VA, Healing the Doctor-Patient Relationship

In opening a dialogue with a veteran, a Syrian American physician is able to overcome prejudices and create a path toward healing.

Raya Elfadel Kheirbek

The man's voice over the phone was angry: "The VA provides terrible care!" I had promised the Veterans Affairs (VA) Medical Center's Patient Advocate Office that I would connect with the man, Mr. Davis, who had called three times before to complain about his care. I was warned beforehand that he was displeased, to say the least.

Volume 36, Number 10. October 2017.
Editor's Note: Patient and clinician names in this essay have been changed.

With him on the line, I took a deep breath and began to look up his records. "I am sorry to hear this, Mr. Davis," I said. "Would you please tell me specifically what is bothering you? I am covering for your doctor and will do my best to help."

Mr. Davis needed to have an MRI for his right shoulder, as was recommended by his military doctor before he separated from the service. He also was having back pain and wasn't exercising enough. He had gained 20 pounds in six months and asked if we offered liposuction.

He had met his primary care clinician, Dr. Kumar, for the first time a couple of weeks earlier and was very uncomfortable when he saw her. To him, there was great insensitivity in the VA's decision to assign him a doctor who he believed was originally from the Middle East.

"Those people wanted to kill me," he remarked to me on the phone, "and I do not appreciate having a doctor who is one of them."

"If you had a woman who was subjected to repeated rape, would you let her be examined by a male doctor?" he continued.

I knew that our policy would allow him to switch doctors, but I had no idea what to say. I had been practicing medicine for a couple of decades and naturally had encountered many types of unusual behavior. Yet I had never heard this type of comment from a patient. I composed myself and quietly explained to Mr. Davis that Dr. Kumar's family came from India. Dr. Kumar herself was born and raised in Pennsylvania and had no connection to the Middle East whatsoever.

But Mr. Davis was insistent on having a doctor who looked like him.

And he was angry.

"I am not your typical patient," he fired back. "I am smart, educated, and highly trained. I do not need your opinion. I have lived in my body for three decades. I know what I want, and your job is to deliver."

He thought the VA worked from nine to five only and found this distressing. When I offered him the possibility of a Saturday appointment, he didn't want it. I offered him early morning appointments, but he said his wife worked as well, and someone needed to walk their dog. He refused to call and make an appointment for the MRI, explaining that he had called a couple of times in the past, and no one had picked up the phone.

I told him that I wanted to meet with him to help resolve these issues and blocked off an hour the following week to meet during my administrative time. He was excited that I would be able to see him quickly, given what he referred to as the long wait time to get an appointment in the VA. He added that, based on our conversation, I seemed to be a good doctor. I gave him my contact information and told him to call if he needed to make any changes before our appointment.

While I was determined to meet and help Mr. Davis, a potential challenge loomed. I am of Middle Eastern origin. I wondered if I should reveal this information after coordinating his care and give him another opportunity to seek a different clinician. My colleagues advised me to stand tall and not give him that choice. To them, his views represented bigotry.

Yet Mr. Davis was not the only one struggling with the past. For me, encountering Mr. Davis brought back painful memories and forced me to stop and reflect on my years of service in the VA, my belief system, and my biases. I wondered if his "bigotry" was really so alien to the human nature in us all.

An Occupational Hazard

As a primary care physician working in the VA, I have heard countless stories from soldiers reliving their experiences in war zones. As an Arab American immigrant, I had followed the Iraq War and—later—the promising start of the Arab Spring and then watched them both spiral into the chaos of death and destruction, including a civil war in my native country, Syria. I felt privileged to be a physician and an American, especially as violence took hold overseas. I could have been back home along with everyone I worried about.

I could be dead. Feeling powerless, I forced myself to watch and listen to the news. The least I could do was to be aware.

On a July morning in 2006, some time before war would break out in my home country, I was driving to work and listening to NPR's *Morning Edition*. The station featured a story about a 14-year-old girl named Abeer, who had lived with her family near a checkpoint in al-Mahmudiyah, Iraq, an area that was then known as the triangle of death. Four armed young American soldiers had stormed into Abeer's house and shot her mother, father, and five-year-old sister. Abeer was taken to an adjacent room in the house where she was gang-raped and murdered, and her body was set on fire. Hearing about this crime sent chills down my spine. I parked my car on the side of the road, cried, and whispered a prayer for this family and for peace.

Later that day I found myself searching for Abeer's story on the internet during my lunch break. The four American soldiers had been arrested. As I read, I caught sight of Abeer's citizenship identification card issued by the Iraqi government, which had an eerie familiarity. My eyes welled up, and I kept clearing my throat as if I was choking on my own guts.

When I got home later that day, I rushed to the basement and searched in a box containing childhood documents I had brought with me when I immigrated to the United States 25 years before. I found my own citizenship identification card, issued by the Syrian government. The little girl in the photo looked exactly like Abeer. I put the photos next to each other and stared in disbelief. That night, I did not sleep. I followed her story closely, and for several months Abeer's horrible fate clouded my mind every time I met a young soldier who had been on active military duty in Iraq.

When I spoke with them during visits, many of the returning soldiers recounted sad and violent scenes from what they called a never-ending war. Many were torn between being with their comrades and being with their families. The majority had symptoms of post-traumatic stress disorder (PTSD) after experiencing continuous fear for their lives, participating in killings, and watching others be killed. None of the patients I treated wanted to be called a hero. None spoke of the supposed triumph or grandeur of war. Many did not even care who won; they just needed and wanted the war to end. My patients talked about fighting an elusive enemy that led them to proclaim an open war on all Iraqis.

It was very difficult for me to listen to their stories. I found myself asking questions about their deployments and what specifically they had done. While I felt a deep appreciation for patients who opened up and talked, I questioned my motive in asking all these questions. To this day, I do not know if my questions came out of a simple curiosity, the desire to provide thorough medical care, or condemnation.

In a staff meeting, I asked my primary care colleagues how they approached the narratives of their patients. Many confided that, given all of the mandated medical screens we had to perform and other time constraints, they could not afford to listen, even if they wanted to.

"It is best to think of their PTSD as an occupational hazard, check the suicide screen, and link the patient with mental health [care]," one colleague said. "They can deal with all that stuff."

In the VA system, after all, we are privileged to have mental health services integrated with primary care, so that a psychologist and a psychiatrist are physically located within the primary care service area and can see patients the same day if needed. My primary care colleagues who did ask questions about their patients' military service histories and made time to listen often found their workweek significantly extended. Many worked long hours on weekends just to keep up.

Listening to my patients' stories took a toll on me. I was afraid to admit or share my feelings with my boss, mentors, or even my family. I did not want anyone to throw doubts on my capability as a physician to treat all people equally. I started searching the medical literature for information on doctors' biases in the aftermath of war and found only one article, in the *British Medical Journal*. It centered on a Jewish surgeon at a German hospital who walked out of the operating room and refused to operate on a patient after spotting a tattoo on his arm of an imperial eagle perched on a swastika. The 46-year-old surgeon, who worked at a hospital in the city of Paderborn, explained later that his conscience prevented him from treating people he suspected of having neo-Nazi sympathies.

There was another reason why I didn't open up about my feelings: I was mortified at the thought that I could be viewed as less than American. I recalled my interview at the US embassy in Damascus early one August afternoon in 1991, after I had applied for a student visa. My friends told me never to say that I would stay in America, as my chances of getting a visa would be better if I said my goal was to train to become a skilled physician so I could come back and serve my fellow Syrian citizens. After several hours of waiting outside the embassy doors on a hot summer day, I had my interview. Through a small window, an embassy employee spoke to me in broken Arabic: "You are a beautiful young woman. How do we know you would not travel to America, fall in love, and stay there?"

I was nervous, spoke little English, and forgot all I was told.

"I sure hope I do," I quickly responded.

He smiled, asked me to wait for a few minutes, and came back. My passport had been stamped with an approved visa. That day and in the days since, I learned that America stood not only for freedom, but also for unconditional love and the freedom to defend that love.

Despite the difficult stories of war I often hear at the VA, my love for this country and commitment to my work never faltered. Years after I had heard Abeer's story, the acuteness of my feelings diminished.

I decided to take up running. Eventually, I was running 10 miles twice a week. I kept pushing myself, dedicating every run to a cause I believed in. I stopped working on weekends and spent more time with my husband—I did fall in love and made a home here, after all—

and our children. I began to feel connected to a normal life outside of a war zone, and I reinforced this connection by avoiding the news after work.

Meeting Mr. Davis

I introduced myself to Mr. Davis on a Tuesday in March 2017, less than a week after our initial phone conversation. A white man in his early 30s, he was tall and well built, with a rectangular face; a defined, slightly pointed chin; and a sturdy jawline. He had light brown hair, small blue eyes, and a straight nose. The jacket he wore over his broad shoulders had neatly polished buttons and was slightly frayed in places. Part of his right hand was missing. He glanced at me with a smile. I am a white woman with green eyes and brown hair.

"I am very happy you were able to make it to this meeting," I said with a big smile.

He nodded in silence and avoided making eye contact.

"I had a chance to review your chart. I think I can help with your physical needs," I added. "But I am also suspecting there are mental health issues that might need to be addressed."

Given his sentiments about Middle Eastern doctors, I thought he had a plausible PTSD diagnosis. When I began to suggest as much, he cut me off.

"This is all stereotyping," he asserted. "I did what I was supposed to do. I will heal through going back to work and being productive."

I caught him looking at my name badge.

"I understand," I said. "Thank you for clarifying."

I asked how he had ended up in the military. He said he'd signed up simply because college was "so damn expensive." He was not a "military brat" and didn't enlist out of a sense of obligation. He was not angry or in need of some form of revenge. It's not that he felt enlisting was brave or important.

"I just needed help with college money," he said. "In retrospect, I could have done something that did not risk being shot at every day."

He broke into a sorrowful smile.

I told him I wanted to be able to help him and needed to know more. I asked about how he'd ended up with his shoulder injury.

Mr. Davis had been in three combat deployments—Iraq in 2010 and Afghanistan in 2011 and 2013—as a member of the US Army Special Forces. He'd been involved in multiple close-range blasts, traumatic jumps, and firefights. Many of the people he had served with had been killed. Since his return to the United States, he had been having constant pain in his right shoulder. He had nightmares one or two times a week, and recently they'd become more frequent. There was one nightmare in particular in which he saw himself collecting the body parts of his dead friends and putting the pieces in a body bag. They had no faces, but somehow he knew they were his friends. He avoided thinking about what had happened over there and avoided talking about it with his friends.

"Few Americans have served," he explained, looking out the window. "I was afraid that I would be judged as a monster or celebrated as a hero."

Nowadays, he said, he attempted to fill his time by working on his master's degree in economics and with other distractions. His wife had told him that he was distant, but he said, she respected his isolation and assumed he needed time to himself.

"What kept you going during all the deployments?" I asked.

"I closed my eyes while hiding from fire and remembered family trips skiing with my little sister and laughing on the slopes of Jackson Hole." He looked up and smiled. I saw a glimpse of the little boy in his face and knew he was in pain. I wanted to reach out and touch his hand, but I was afraid he would not welcome my gesture.

"Have you had thoughts of hurting yourself or others?" I asked.

"No. My friend did." He paused for a moment. "He was long dead before he pulled the trigger. I myself sleep with my gun at my side but [have] never used it."

I asked if he'd had any good experiences in Iraq.

Yes, he said. It touched him to see families with young children walking for many miles to collect American parachutes to help build houses. The local people found something useful to do with even the trash that Americans had left. All his memories, however, were haunted by the killings he had witnessed and the poverty of the places he had been.

Mr. Davis had seen mental health providers during his active service, but he did not feel like elaborating on that for me. We discussed his back and shoulder pain. While examining him, I noticed a tattoo on his left arm: the word *kafer* (meaning infidel) written in Arabic. For a split second, I considered telling him that I could read this, but I held my tongue. I'll admit in retrospect that I was a bit scared of him.

We scheduled an MRI appointment, and then Mr. Davis told me about some numbness in his injured hand. An improvised explosive device had detonated in his hand while he was clearing an insurgent field in Fallujah, he explained. I referred him to a hand surgeon. We decided to draw labs and reevaluate his condition in a week.

I felt it was then time to address his comments about Dr. Kumar. I said: "You know, Mr. Davis, you are a man of tremendous courage. It is not easy to share your experiences with someone else, especially experiences of this nature."

He looked out the window.

"You mentioned to me in our phone conversation last week that you were uncomfortable with a doctor from the Middle East."

I paused, and then continued. "I want you to be comfortable, and I am very happy we met today. I want to thank you for allowing me into your life and for the opportunity to help. I owe to you the knowledge that I was born and raised in Syria."

The few seconds of silence that ensued felt like an eternity.

Then Mr. Davis abruptly got to his feet and raised his severed hand. "I am so sorry I was being a jerk. I would really like you to be my physician—unless you do not feel comfortable caring for me, based on my earlier comments."

I stood up and extended my hand to him. "It was important for us to talk. Please keep doing so, as it's the only way for us to deal with such emotions."

His face broke out into a wide smile. He was absolutely thrilled at the prospect of us working together. I was too.

Healing Takes Time

Though I have served in the VA for many years and in different roles, my focus has always been on patients. The sacred time spent with patients in an exam room is the only lasting truth in medicine. In this large bureaucratic system, all else can wait. Yet many priorities compete for our attention during a single visit. It might not be possible to spend the needed time on each important issue. While a slew of mandatory screenings for diseases has improved our medical care, it is equally crucial to take the time to develop a relationship with the patient, exploring his or her service history and the lived experiences that may come with that. It is not always easy. In my work, I know what it is like to be discriminated against, and what it is like to have stereotypes of my own. Yet an admission of our own vulnerability and opening the door to a conversation about self-care, compassion, understanding, and human connection is how we attend to all aspects of our patients' suffering—and perhaps some of our own.

With the implementation of the Veterans Access, Choice, and Accountability Act of 2014, our VA patients now have the option to seek medical care in the private sector as well as through the VA, so it becomes even more important than ever to ensure the existence of a broad system of caring that addresses their complex physical and psychological needs. It is only then that true healing can begin.

When Patients Mentor Doctors

The Story of One Vital Bond

A physician reconnects with the patient who mentored her as a medical student and helps him make a final care decision.

Aroonsiri Sangarlangkarn

It was a cold December morning in 2015, and Roger was slowly dying. With end-stage chronic obstructive pulmonary disease (COPD), Roger had been in and out of the hospital for months, each episode worse than the last. Once a functional New Yorker who walked to his favorite corner store with an oxygen tank, Roger had morphed into a gaunt skeleton, tethered to his bed by entangling tubes and masks. Time was precious as death closed in, and Roger was wasting it in a lonely, restrictive hospital room.

"He's not going to hospice," my nurse practitioner told me during inpatient rounds. "We talked to him, and he didn't want to hear any of it."

"Let me try," I offered.

"Best of luck," she said with a sigh. "He's not the easiest to talk to."

"I know," I said, taking a deep breath. "I know him from before."

Then I went to talk to Roger—my patient, my friend.

The First Time We Met

Roger and I met during my first year as a medical student at the Icahn School of Medicine at Mount Sinai in New York City on the first day of the school's Seniors as Mentors Program. For four years, students were paired with patients ages 65 and older who volunteered to teach us about medicine from a patient's perspective. They allowed us to accompany them to doctor visits, explore their health in the

Volume 36, Number 3. March 2017.
Editor's Note: The patient's last name was omitted to protect his privacy.

home, and get to know them outside of the hospital setting. It promised to be a memorable relationship, and I was excited to see what my patient mentor would be like.

I waded through the hectic meeting hall filled with a sea of very old patients and very young medical students to find Roger, a gentleman barely older than age 65 with salt-and-pepper hair and a portable oxygen tank. After 40 years of smoking, he had lost one lung to cancer while the other succumbed to severe emphysema. Through pursed lips and wheezes escaping from his diseased airways, he offered a labored hello as we shook hands.

Roger possessed an odd combination of traits: He was extremely intelligent with great attention to detail, but he was also eccentric in a way that could be off-putting. He would impress me with his extensive knowledge of Thailand, my home country, but in the next breath he would call me "Oriental," an outdated phrase that made me feel like a physical object from the East. We would have long discussions about the marvels of the internet, and then he would incessantly email me with requests for Facebook friendship, a gesture that made me feel uneasy. When Roger told me that he did not have many friends and that he was estranged from his brother, the only family he had left, I partly understood why. Sometimes at doctor appointments, his obsession with detail and his social oddities would unfold into awkward arguments with doctors about the minute particulars of various treatment plans. Most of these conversations ended with a frustrated provider and Roger asking for more time to process his options.

Although I got to know intimate details of Roger's life through the mentoring program, I struggled, even in my own mind, to clearly define my relationship with him. Because of his age and his awkward quirks, I did not think of Roger as a friend, and because I was not his doctor, I did not think of him as a patient. It would not be until years later, after I had patients of my own, that I truly understood the gravity of my medical school experience with him.

The Man Who Loved "Go"

Several years later at Mount Sinai, I was finishing up a fellowship in geriatrics when an attending physician flagged me down in our clinic.

"Hey, I think you know one of my patients," the physician said. "You took a really detailed social history of him a few years ago."

That patient was Roger. At the physician's request, we looked at Roger's medical chart together and discussed his case before going in to see him. Having seen many impersonal, uninformative patient records by that point, I was reminded of how insightful a medical history can be when written by someone who really knows the patient. In my student notes from several years ago, I'd written down the names of Roger's parents and where he was born. I'd told a story of how he grew up in the Presbyterian Church and how his skepticism of it led him to become an atheist. I'd described how he always dreamed of being an architect as a boy and talked about what England was like when he designed buildings there in 1972. I'd even gone into great detail about how Roger played Go, a Chinese board game, probably because I liked the game myself and we used to have long conversations about it. Years of stories came flooding back through the notes, and I remembered Roger.

I remembered him despite the new long white beard he'd grown and the bald spots where his salt-and-pepper hair used to be. He remembered me, too, even with a new haircut and a long white coat. Despite our changed appearances, our connection was the same: Roger was still the elderly, intellectual man who loved Go, and I was still the girl from Thailand who worked in the same New York hospital.

A Different Kind of Friendship

Soon after I happened upon Roger in the clinic, his COPD began to worsen, and he started coming to the hospital frequently with

COPD exacerbations. During the first visit, he recovered well enough to return home. But after a few admissions, it was clear that his body was failing him, and the likelihood of Roger returning to the walk-up apartment where he lived alone was getting slim.

As fate would have it, I got to be one of the doctors who took care of Roger during these admissions. Of all the health professionals on his team, I was the only person who had a chance to visit Roger at home. No one knew how Roger navigated the oxygen tubing covering his apartment floor but me, and I began to recognize the significance of getting to know patients beyond the incomplete picture we saw in the hospital. To effectively provide care for someone, it's important to learn who they are, what they eat, how they breathe. Being able to visit patients in their homes is the first stage in building this crucial understanding, and this was true for Roger as it was for other patients I had visited at home. However, with Roger I was able to take the second step of building a relationship with him over the years, and this bond would prove helpful to our medical team during Roger's inpatient stay. Since he often grew skeptical when discussing treatment details with unfamiliar providers, I became the designated communicator for the team. It was a privilege I welcomed; after reporting the chest X-ray findings of the day, I would sit by Roger's bed and talk New York politics with him.

Telling a Friend He Is Dying

When it was clear that Roger's remaining lung was quickly deteriorating, I went to tell my friend that he was dying.

I walked into his room with my usual greeting, trying in vain to convince myself that this conversation would be the same as delivering bad news to any other patient. We talked about the weather, and I asked permission to discuss the medical updates of the day. When I told him his lung was getting worse, he said he knew.

"What's next?" he asked. I took a deep breath to brace myself for what was next.

"I can't imagine how hard this must be for you to hear, because this is extremely difficult for me to say." I reached for his hand and grabbed it. "Since we've known each other for so many years . . ."

Roger squeezed my hand, and I started to sob uncontrollably. My last shred of composure gave way to waves of overwhelming sorrow. It was hard to tell my friend that he was dying, that I could not save him.

"How long?" Roger asked. I could hear the trepidation in his voice.

"Less than six months," I answered, my voice shaken by guilt and the feeling of failure.

"I think I've heard enough for today," he said after a long silence. "But I'm glad you're the one who came to tell me."

The Road to Hospice

By that cold December morning in 2015, about a week after I told Roger he was dying, a few providers had tried to offer hospice to him, unsuccessfully. Knowing him and understanding what was important to him, I knew that Roger would logically pick hospice if he could get past his mistrust and concerns over the details. Here was my chance to help guide Roger through one of the most important decisions of his life, and I did not want to fail.

"I know I can't fix your lungs," I started, cautiously choosing my words, "but I am going to make sure that you are always comfortable, no matter what happens."

He nodded calmly.

I pressed on: "I want to make sure that you will always have help when breathing becomes more difficult, and the best place to keep you comfortable is at inpatient hospice."

I paused for his reaction.

"OK," Roger answered, his reply slow and contemplative. "What you're saying makes sense."

I could sense him letting down his guard, relinquishing the skepticism he had toward unfamiliar providers in prior hospice conversations. With relief, sadness, and hope—all embedded in a single question—he asked, "Where is inpatient hospice?"

I squeezed his hands. Roger was ready.

Innovations in Patient-Centered Care

With a growing number of physicians working in shifts, shorter resident duty-hour limits, and a greater demand on physicians to work in specialized fields, patient care is increasingly fragmented, involving multiple handoffs with multiple doctors. According to a 2010 survey conducted by the market research firm GfK, of 1,035 adults in the United States, patients reported seeing an average of 18.7 different doctors during their lives. The numbers were even higher for poorer and older adults (who reported seeing 22.4 and 28.4 doctors during their lives, respectively).

With more handoffs, the therapeutic relationship gets weakened, for both the patient and the provider. According to a 2009 *Archives of Internal Medicine* article, 75 percent of patients in a Chicago hospital could not name a single physician in charge of their care. This is potentially associated with suboptimal care: a small 2001 study published in the *Mayo Clinic Proceedings* reported that correctly identifying photos of physician caregivers was significantly associated with a patient's satisfaction with physician responsiveness and style of addressing questions regarding medical care.

When patients refuse to repeat the story of why they came into the hospital for yet another new provider, I empathize with them. As a geriatrics fellow in the hospital, I usually see patients after they have already talked to emergency medicine residents, emergency medicine attending physicians, surgical consultants, night-float residents, internal medicine residents, medical students, a handful of nurses, and numerous patient care associates. When patients appear skeptical after hearing our medical recommendations, I empathize with them, too. I'd also be skeptical if I didn't know the name of the person recommending the next major step in my care.

Roger was not my peer, and we never did become Facebook friends. But once I became a physician with patients of my own, I grew to understand that Roger and I had a different kind of friendship. After following him for many years, a few times into his home, I knew Roger beyond his COPD, and he knew me beyond my white coat. Understanding how he made decisions, I presented Roger with a single treatment choice that was in line with his values and avoided the inherent skepticism he felt when processing detailed health care options. When listening to my medical recommendations, Roger not only had the advantage of knowing my name—he also had gotten to know me outside the hospital doors and developed a kind of trust from our years of friendship.

For physicians, the ability to learn about our patients' lives beyond the traditional care settings is invaluable. It creates an irreplaceable understanding of patients as people and a powerful trust that can overcome barriers in health care. Yet our ability to connect with patients on a meaningful level is challenged constantly. In medical school, we are taught to apply the same script to every patient, regardless of who they are: start every visit by asking about the chief complaint, describe every patient beginning with their age and sex. In clinics, visits are becoming shorter to achieve higher productivity, and billing and chart documentation barely leave any time for meaningful conversations. Our interactions with patients have become so regimented and one-dimensional that we no longer get to know the multifaceted person outside the hospital.

As we struggle to provide continuity of care despite multiple hand-offs, to recreate the joy of medicine amidst increasing burnout, and to promote a patient-centered approach to health care, the answer to all three may lie in encouraging longitudinal relationships built equally in the health care setting and in the patient's home. This can begin, as it did in my case, during medical training. A number of US medical schools currently offer senior mentor programs similar to the one I participated in, in which medical students are paired with older patients to learn about health care through the lens of the geriatric population. The innovation, initially sponsored by the John A. Hartford Foundation and the Association of American Medical Colleges, included programs such as the University of South Carolina School of Medicine's Senior Mentor Program, launched in 2000. Such programs should be expanded to include patients of all ages and should be offered to physicians and nonphysician health professionals alike.

In real-world practice, home visits should be incentivized, as they can create relational continuity and provide tremendous information on patients' lives outside the hospital. For example, a 2016 study from Norway, published in the journal *Midwifery*, reported that postpartum women experienced a sense of "predictability, availability, and confidence" when visited at home in the postpartum period by midwives who were present during birth.

Once the critical provider-patient bond develops, our health care system must provide an infrastructure to ensure that bond can flourish and support patients across all care settings. I was involved in Roger's hospital admissions out of sheer luck, but that should not be the norm. During transitions or hospital admissions, care should always be coordinated with a designated provider, someone on the patient's care team who has established trust and understanding of the patient over a longitudinal relationship. This designated provider may be an oncologist for a cancer patient or a social worker for an at-risk youth. They might not always need to participate in day-to-day care, but as consultants they can help guide patients through challenging medical situations or coordinate care during transitions. Mobile health technology might help maintain these valuable connections if logistics or limited resources prohibit face-to-face interactions.

The Last Handoff

On another cold morning later in the month, I met up with Ben, the hospice liaison, to ensure a smooth care transition for Roger. We discussed the details of his care, and I told Ben everything I knew about the man who loved Go.

"Your name carried a lot of weight with him," Ben said. "You must have known each other a long time."

"Since I was a medical student," I answered, as fond memories came rushing back. "I'm glad I got to take care of him. He doesn't really have a friend to advocate for him."

"Well, he does," Ben replied. "You are his friend."

5

Disparities and Discrimination

- "Go Back to California": When Providers Fail
  Transgender Patients *Laura Arrowsmith*

- A Simple Case of Chest Pain: Sensitizing Doctors to Patients
  with Disabilities *Leana S. Wen*

- Grasping at the Moon: Enhancing Access to Careers in the
  Health Professions *Louis W. Sullivan*

- Bridging the Divide between Dental and Medical Care
  Gayathri Subramanian

- In Rural Towns, Immigrant Doctors Fill a Critical Need
  Yasmin Sokkar Harker

- An Uninsured Immigrant Delays Needed Care *Cheryl Bettigole*

"Go Back to California"

When Providers Fail Transgender Patients

A transgender doctor is mistreated by a health care provider—and wants to make the system better for patients like her.

Laura Arrowsmith

Go back to California, the physician at a minor emergency center in a suburb of Tulsa, Oklahoma, told me. The words were flung—practically vomited—at me. I had gone to the center, a relatively new building that was beautifully decorated, on a Sunday morning in 2010 in terrible pain due to complications from a previous surgery. The receptionist was pleasant, and the physician had entered the exam room smiling. He was about 50 years old and seemed friendly. But when I explained why I was there, the friendly smile quickly disappeared, and his face contorted into an expression of disgust and revulsion.

Two days earlier I had returned to Tulsa from a week-long stay in California, where I had undergone a secondary labiaplasty—a procedure that refines the shape of the inner labia of the vagina. For this procedure, I had returned to the surgeon who performed my original genital reassignment surgery in 2005, confident that she could make some minor improvements. She was one of the leading specialists in the world, a gynecologist who herself had traveled the same medical journey as me, from male sex assigned at birth to female. After returning home from this second surgery, I had developed a minor abscess around one suture. It was extremely painful and terribly frightening. I lived more than a thousand miles from where the surgeon practiced, and my family practice physician was not available on the weekend. Hence, the demoralizing and disastrous weekend visit to the minor emergency center.

Volume 36, Number 9. September 2017.

The doctor's words reverberated in my head: "Go back to California." He fled the exam room soon after he'd uttered them, without examining me or obtaining any further history.

I was devastated, angry, scared, embarrassed . . . and ashamed. It wasn't the first time a physician had made me—also a physician—feel this way. And it's a problem in health care that simply must change.

Living "Like a Girl"

I am a transgender woman, meaning that I was identified at birth as male, but I have known since my earliest memories that I am a woman. When I was growing up in small-town Kansas during the 1950s and 1960s, there was no internet, and there were no books, television shows, or other media that could have affirmed for me that I was not the only person who felt this way.

For many Americans, life was easier, simpler, and less cluttered during the decades of my childhood. For me, that was not the case. My only sibling, a younger sister, was my main playmate before my school years began. We played with dolls—dress-up and paper—during the day when my father wasn't around. I learned quickly that in the evenings when he was home, it had to be trucks and toy guns, cowboys and Indians. He was the gender police for me.

"You walk like a girl," he would tell me. Or, you throw a ball like a girl. You stand like a girl. You get dressed like a girl. You blow your nose like a girl (yes, he said even that). These were behaviors that were to be eliminated. I quickly learned to be ashamed of the woman inside me and became fearful of showing any suggestion of femininity lest I be punished. At night, I would pray for God to let me wake up as a girl, but I intuitively knew that I could share my true feelings with no one else. My father was never physically abusive, but he was an intimidating presence not to be crossed or disappointed.

Suppression and denial became my daily ritual. I spent decades living as society expected me to do, and hid "her" (my true self) behind a veneer of masculinity. I went to college and medical school to become an osteopathic physician. I got married and helped raise four children.

Yet in moments when I found myself alone, I would put on women's clothing. It just felt so right. I would look at myself in a mirror and be so disappointed in the reflection. Sometimes I "borrowed" a few items of my wife's clothing. When I could, I purchased my own feminine clothes, carefully hidden to put on in private moments. Eventually, I would promise myself I would never dress up that way again. I would discard my treasured clothing in some place where it would never be discovered. This cycle repeated itself endlessly.

This emotional turmoil is common and is known as "gender dysphoria." In some trans people, the disorder may be accompanied by substance abuse, self-harm, or eating disorders as a means of coping with the tremendous pain that is experienced. Forty percent will attempt suicide.

By the time I was in my 50s, my gender dysphoria—which previously would strike me for a period of unbearable hours, days, or even weeks but then would pass—had become constant. The condition was there when I awoke and lasted until I fell asleep. It was like a car alarm I was powerless to silence.

One afternoon I parked my truck in a parking lot next to a busy four-lane street. I got out of the truck and watched as a large red semi headed my way. I walked in front of it, hoping my death might be viewed as an accident. The driver managed to swerve away from me, somehow, and I was unharmed. The next thing I remember, I was walking back to my truck. I sat inside and cried and cried. It was then I knew that I had to find help. Soon.

By then, with the advent of the internet, I was able to learn more about what I was feeling. In time, I found websites with credible information. One of the first things I learned was that there was a word for people like me: transgender. Soon I found other websites that provided information that likely saved my life—lists of mental health therapists who provided therapeutic support for transgender people and information about successful hormonal and surgical treatments that could enable me to become my true self. Finally, I had hope. I found an online support group of transgender women at various stages in their journeys: They were happy, beautiful, and alive. Over the next few months, I was able to connect with some of them by telephone and in person. At last I had found the path to becoming who I felt myself to be. I ran down that path and never looked back.

Gender Identity Is Hardwired

Gender identity—that internal sense of knowing oneself to be a man, woman, or nonbinary—is understood to typically be fully developed by around the age of four years, sometimes even earlier. Gender identity is unchanging and unchangeable, hardwired into our brains. All of us inherently know our gender identity: it is not a conscious decision but rather one aspect of everything that makes each of us an individual. A transgender person is simply born with a gender identity that does not match that person's body.

Research has shown that being transgender is most likely due to a hormonal imbalance in utero that happens during the period of a pregnancy when the fetal brain is differentiating into a male or female brain. Autopsy studies, functional MRI scans, and SPECT (single-photon emission computed tomography) scans suggest that some people are born with a male brain and a female body, or vice versa. (Male and female brains have been shown to be slightly different in structure.) These studies suggest that transgender people have the brains that match their gender identities even before taking any cross-sex hormones.

It should be noted that not all of the people who identify as transgender feel themselves to be of the opposite sex. The 2015 US Transgender Discrimination Survey of approximately 28,000 trans people showed that many respondents identified themselves variously as gender nonbinary, androgynous, gender nonconforming, gender queer, gender fluid, or agender. Younger generations are moving beyond the idea that one must live in the world with a strictly binary (male or female) gender identity.

A lot has changed. During my childhood, teen, and even adult years, transgender people were viewed as defective. Attempts to cure what was viewed as deviant behavior or mental illness included electroshock therapy, massive hormone doses, intense psychotherapy, and psychiatric hospitalization. Aversion therapy, which attempted to replace "maladaptive" with "normal" behavior through a system of negative stimuli and rewards, was advocated. None of these treatments were effective in treating transgender children, teens, and adults. Research and clinical experience gradually demonstrated that it is not efficacious to attempt to "fix" the brain; rather, it is effective to provide medical and surgical treatment (if desired) to change the body to conform with and affirm a person's gender identity.

When I began my journey to become my authentic self, my family practice physician of many years refused to see me. She said that I had lied to her about who I was. This was a shock—but then, I guess I had lied to myself for decades too. On numerous other occasions I have been refused care by physicians, sometimes due to discrimination and bigotry, but at other times due to an expressed concern that "we have no idea how to care for a transgender patient."

A 2010 Lambda Legal study showed that 50 percent of transgender patients who were fortunate enough to find a physician who would care for them had to teach the physician what to do. Providing sensitive medical care to transgender patients should be relatively straightforward. Multiple organizations such as the Endocrine Society and the World Professional Association for Transgender Health (WPATH) provide online protocols for this type of medical care. The July 2016 issue of the *Journal of Family Practice* also published a fairly comprehensive article outlining ways to provide sensitive care to transgender patients.

But because so few physicians will treat this population, many transgender people have given up trying to find medical care or are afraid to seek routine and emergency care. A January 2014 Williams

Institute study on transgender suicidality showed that 60 percent of transgender patients who, because of antitransgender bias, are unable to find physicians who will provide medical care for them have attempted suicide.

Fortunately, after several years, I finally found a family practice physician who is accepting and open-minded. I was the first transgender patient she had treated, so I have had to educate her about our treatment, follow-up care, and culture. She has proved to be a wonderful learner.

Appropriate treatment for transgender patients, as outlined by the WPATH standards of care, includes supportive mental health counseling to deal with the emotional turmoil created by years of dealing with the body-soul-brain mismatch. Medical treatment includes hormonal therapy to feminize the male body or masculinize the female one. Various sophisticated surgeries can be performed to do the same thing. Numerous professional organizations, including the American Medical Association, have issued policy statements to the effect that gender affirmation surgery is medically necessary for the treatment of gender dysphoria.

It should be noted, however, that most transgender people do not choose gender-affirming surgeries. One common reason is a lack of insurance coverage. Many patients have no financial ability to pay for any medical care. Such treatment also may be contraindicated because of a co-occurring medical issue. Still others choose not to transition out of fear of loss of employment, family, extended family, or friends.

Unfortunately, information about the appropriate treatment for transgender patients has not been taught in medical schools or postgraduate programs until recently, and even now it is only infrequently included in the basic few hours of LGBT education that the schools and programs provide. Most physicians currently in practice have no training in how to care for transgender people.

In fact, several studies, including those by Lambda Legal and the National Center for Transgender Equality, have consistently shown that there is extensive discrimination in health care directed toward transgender patients, including the refusal of medical care, the provision of incorrect care, and verbal or physical abuse by physicians.

There is a critical need for state and federal transgender antidiscrimination legislation to ensure not only employment rights—the focus of most current efforts—but also the right to competent medical care, housing, and education.

Not Uncommon

After being refused medical care for my acute abscess at the minor emergency center, I was able to tolerate the pain until my family practice physician could drain the abscess and provide antibiotics. I healed physically without further difficulty, but the emotional scars from this event and countless others remain. When I meet a new physician for the first time, I automatically anticipate rejection or discrimination—or at the very least, the need to educate the physician about the transgender population, the proper terminology to use, and what constitutes appropriate care.

During medical school, my peers and I were taught about obscure medical diseases, conditions that I never saw during my 30-plus years of medical practice. Many of these were covered multiple times and in a variety of classes. Transgender patients, in contrast, are not uncommon. Every practicing physician will encounter transgender patients in his or her practice. Yet medical education in the United States is failing to teach medical students and residents how to care for this population. This has to change. No patient meeting a physician for the first time should fear being denied care or given incorrect treatment. The expression on a caring professional's face should be one of concern and interest, not a snarl of angry disgust.

A Simple Case of Chest Pain

Sensitizing Doctors to Patients with Disabilities

A doctor who stutters confronts the stigma against patients—and providers—with disabilities.

Leana S. Wen

It was midnight in the emergency department (ED), and the senior resident, Stan, was on a roll. Clad in green scrubs two sizes too small for his body to emphasize his muscular physique, he dashed between the ambulance bay and the critical care rooms.

"Wen!" he barked at me, the intern. "Come over here to do the 'rule-out heart attack' in three." Two medical students grabbed their notepads and followed Stan and me into the room.

The patient did not look as if he was having a heart attack. Dressed in a tailored suit, the young man with a neat ponytail sat in bed, texting on his BlackBerry. The nurse's note said the 31-year-old was having chest pain. His vital signs and electrocardiogram were normal.

"Good evening!" boomed Stan. We formed an imposing circle around the stretcher. "How are you doing?"

"I'm f-f-f-f-ine," the young man said. He looked up at us. "Call me J-J . . . J-J-J-J . . ."

Stan glanced over my shoulder at his chart. "James, right? Do you still have chest pain?"

I dutifully wrote down that the patient appeared in no obvious distress and was breathing normally. But James seemed distressed about something. "N-N-N . . ." he stammered, his eyes looking around the room until they settled resolutely on the ground. His face was red with effort. Sweat pooled around his brows. His brown eyes

Volume 33, Number 10. October 2014.
Editor's Note: The senior resident's name was changed to protect his privacy. The patient, James, asked that his last name be omitted.

swept upward and landed on mine. I gave him an encouraging smile. "N-N-No, I'm g-g-good," he said.

Stan was heading for the door. "Talk to him; I'll put in for labs and a chest X-ray," he called out as he left the room, the students trailing behind. "Oh, and make sure to say things slooooowly so he understands."

By the look on James's face, I could tell that he understood just fine. I did, too. I closed the door. "I'm so sorry," I said. "Let's start over. My name is Leana. I'm your doctor. I'm also a person who stutters."

Hiding My Disability

I wasn't always open about being a person who stutters. In fact, it took me 22 years to admit to myself that I stuttered and needed treatment for it. From an early age, I knew that I had trouble getting out my words, but after seeing classmates bully other kids for this, I vowed never to let my disfluency show. I became a covert stutterer, hiding my disability using tricks such as avoiding certain words and situations. I could never ask for "water," only "a drink." "Pen" became "something to write with." Once, when giving a talk on the Roman Empire in fourth grade, I was so afraid of stuttering on the word "Roman" that I jabbed a pencil into my thigh so that I would be released from class to see the school nurse. The little piece of lead is still there today.

By the time I went to college, I became so proficient at hiding my stuttering that I rarely revealed it in public. By medical school, it became more difficult to hide. It seemed a cruel irony that I had trouble with the word "doctor" and had to come up with other ways to address my attending physicians. During an infectious disease lecture, I was called on to answer a question. With the spotlight on, I could not get out the word for a particular disease caused by parasitic worms—"schistosomiasis"—and there was no appropriate substitute. "Sch-sch-sch," the professor imitated, shaking his head. "Why don't you come back when you learn to speak?" His sharp words, like the broken piece of pencil lead, will always stay with me.

Through the Looking Glass

As I sat with James in the ED bay, I thought back to the scorn of classmates and professors I faced over the years. "I'm not stupid," James said. He finally looked me in the eyes, and I could see tears gathering. "I just have trouble getting out w-w-w-words sometimes." I sat and talked with him for about 10 minutes. He told me he was a lawyer. He always knew he had a problem with his speech, but, like me, he was able to hide his stuttering most of the time.

Two weeks prior to our meeting in the ED, James had been promoted to a position in his law firm with greater visibility and more demands for communication with clients. The harder he tried to speak fluently, the more struggled his speech became. The evening of his visit to the ED, James had been having dinner with clients when he began to stutter on every other word. He struggled with his speech so much that he began sweating and breathing quickly. His colleagues asked if he was having chest pain, and when he nodded, they called for an ambulance. That is how he ended up sitting on a stretcher in the ED struggling to speak with me.

James didn't need blood work or an X ray, I realized. He needed someone to listen to him. His providers didn't have to be experts on speech disorders, but they needed to have some basic understanding of how to recognize and treat patients who stutter. It's a disorder that affects at least three million Americans, or 1 percent of the population.

While medical school curricula are replete with lectures on "one-in-a-million" diseases, little attention is devoted to teaching future doctors how to care for people with speech disorders or other disabilities. A 2005 special report commissioned by the Special Olympics found that only 25 percent of medical schools included in their curricula any content regarding people with disabilities. A 2012 *Academic Medicine* article by Laurie Woodard and colleagues found little improvement, with accreditation councils still not requiring clinicians to have knowledge of caring for people with disabilities.

Yet, according to the 2010 census, nearly 20 percent of Americans—representing 57 million adults and 5.2 million children—have a disability. The Americans with Disabilities Act (ADA) of 1990 defines a person with disability as someone who has a physical or mental impairment that substantially limits one or more major life activities. The World Health Organization adds that disability is not the physical health condition itself but the limitation experienced because of the health condition in interaction with societal and environmental barriers. Some people are born with their disabilities; others may acquire them through injury, chronic disease, or aging.

Care for the 20 Percent

As we talked, I told James what it was like to go through medical training as a person who stutters and how I saw firsthand the ignorance and prejudice some health care providers harbor toward patients with disabilities. For instance, I remember an attending physician berating me for testing someone with pelvic pain for sexually transmitted diseases. The patient was "wheelchair-bound"; surely she couldn't be sexually active, the attending said. On the wards there were frequent jabs about people disabled from chronic pain—why couldn't they just work like everyone else?

Like James, patients may have had unnecessary tests ordered because of their disability. Doctors and nurses label such practice with the disparaging term of "veterinary medicine." In other words, just as for an animal that can't speak for itself, they order tests instead of talking to patients who are perceived as being "slow" or "difficult." These patients often receive inadequate care: either doctors can't see past their disability and attribute all problems to it, or doctors fail to acknowledge the true impact of their impairments.

Numerous reports have documented that people with disabilities have poorer health and receive inferior health care. According to the National Health Interview Survey, 3.4 percent of adults without disabilities report fair or poor health compared with 30.6 percent of those with difficulty seeing or hearing, 37.9 percent of those with movement difficulties, and 63.8 percent of those with cognitive difficulties. People with disabilities are more likely to be obese, inactive, and smokers, and yet they receive less information on screening and other preventive services.

They also face significant barriers to accessing care. In a 2013 study, Tara Lagu and colleagues described a telephone survey of 256 doctors' offices in four cities. Researchers called the offices to make an appointment for a fictional patient who was obese and paralyzed from the waist down. More than one in five offices stated that they could not accommodate this patient, citing reasons such as lack of trained staff and lack of equipment to transfer the patient from wheelchair to exam table.

As I saw blatant examples of unequal and insensitive care to patients with disabilities, I felt anger, then shame and fear. I knew that the right thing to do was to speak up, but I was so afraid that I would be exposing myself and my own disability. Throughout medical training, my greatest fear was that my supervisors would find out about my stuttering and deem me unfit to fulfill my dream of becoming a doctor. There were few doctors with disabilities to serve as role models. Although one or two of my professors stuttered, they never talked about it. I don't recall anyone else, not a colleague or superior, who was open about having a disability. Numerous studies have reported that physicians harbor negative perceptions of people with disabilities. The stigma is compounded by lack of exposure: two surgeon general reports cite lack of provider training as a major barrier to equitable care for people with disabilities.

Toward a Better Future

James's blood tests and X-ray came back: the results were normal. I went to give him the good news, but he didn't seem relieved.

"I know it's not a heart attack," he said. "But what do I do next time this happens?"

I told James about how speech therapy has helped me address feelings of fear and shame about my disability. Becoming totally fluent isn't the goal of speech therapy—I continue to stutter from time to time. The goal is to say what we want to say without avoiding words or situations. As I gave him his discharge papers, James and I exchanged numbers, and I assured him that I would follow up with information on therapy and support groups in the area.

Improving care for people with disabilities is an ethical imperative. The United Nations Convention on the Rights of Persons with Disabilities affirms that people with disabilities "have the right to the enjoyment of the highest attainable standard of health without discrimination on the basis of disability."

Because nearly every provider will take care of substantial numbers of people with disabilities during his or her career, health professional education must mandate training focused on recognizing and caring for people with disabilities. Some medical schools have started pilot programs. At the University of South Carolina, for instance, a rehabilitation specialist with a spinal cord injury and a family medicine professor with a daughter who has a cognitive impairment teach a 90-minute course for medical students that emphasizes the biopsychosocial context of disabilities. At the University of South Florida, medical students visit community centers, participate in service learning, and interact with patients with disabilities. Subsequent research has shown that both the South Carolina and Florida programs increased students' comfort with and willingness to provide care to people with disabilities.

These early efforts are evidence that early educational programs can work. The Association of American Medical Colleges, the Accreditation Council for Graduate Medical Education, and their osteopathic counterparts should make learning to care for people with disabilities part of the required curriculum. Kristi Kirschner and Raymond Curry proposed six core competencies for medical trainees in a 2009 *Journal of the American Medical Association* article. They suggest, for example, that medical students should demonstrate that they can treat patients who have disabilities with compassion and dignity, and resident physicians should be able to address their patients' acute medical issues.

The Affordable Care Act broadly supports the development of curricula to train health care providers on better care for people with disabilities. This recommendation is a good start, but it needs to be backed by funding to implement a national curriculum for medical, nursing, and other health professional students. By developing interdisciplinary modules and ensuring that people with disabilities are part of every step of the curriculum implementation, such a national curriculum can be a transformative model for patient-centered medical education.

Finally, students with disabilities should be encouraged to enter the medical profession and to educate others about their experiences. Disability rights advocates have long held that doctors with disabilities can deliver safe and effective health care and, in fact, may have advantages in terms of the empathy and communication skills they bring to their work. Medical societies can be proactive about establishing technical standards for each field and can actively recruit a diverse workforce that includes people with disabilities. Health care providers who themselves have disabilities can serve as powerful advocates and begin to counter prevalent biases and stigma.

Acceptance

It took me until the end of medical school to accept my own identity as a person who stutters and to be open about it with others. Talking to people about stuttering and advocating for people with disabilities have been instrumental in my own healing. Now, as an attending, I lecture to health professionals and students about my experiences. I provide advice for how to treat patients with speech impediments. Let them finish their sentences, for example. Look them in the eye, nod, and be encouraging. And speak up when you see someone receiving inadequate care because of their stuttering or other disability.

At the end of my ED shift that night, I asked Stan if we could have a word. We walked to an empty trauma bay. My hands were shaking, and I could hear my own stutter return as I began to explain what was actually going on with James and how Stan's comments hurt him—and me.

There was a long silence when I finished. "Do you have his number?" Stan asked me. I did. To my surprise, he took the number and called James to apologize. Stan then asked me to put together a seminar on disabilities for other trainees in our hospital. In the seminar's first session, medical students and residents began by discussing how they had also witnessed inappropriate behavior toward people with disabilities but were too afraid to speak up.

I invited James to be the inaugural guest lecturer in a series of small-group, patient-led rounds. He talked poignantly about the dynamic nature of disability and about how disability is a human condition that everyone will encounter in his or her lifetime. I've kept in touch with James, and he and I mentor a group of college students who also are people who stutter. Six years later, James is a partner at his law firm and speaks openly about being a lawyer who stutters. He, too, likes to tell the story of how a simple case of chest pain led him to accept his identity and become a mentor, teacher, and advocate.

Grasping at the Moon

Enhancing Access to Careers in the Health Professions

A former Secretary of Health and Human Services reflects on what's needed to enable more minorities to become doctors and other health professionals.

Louis W. Sullivan

When I was a child in our small town of Blakely, Georgia, the seat of Early County, there were only two doctors. Both were white, with separate waiting rooms for their white and black patients. For blacks,

Volume 35, Number 8. August 2016.

this usually meant going around to the back of the building to enter the blacks-only waiting room.

Growing up in rural southwest Georgia in the 1930s, during the Great Depression, I witnessed poverty, poor health, and deprivation firsthand in our community. We lived under a social structure of legally enforced brutal segregation. Blacks could not vote or otherwise participate in government. For employment, they were relegated to lower-paying positions, if they were fortunate enough to have a job at all.

Most black farmers were not landowners; they worked as share-croppers on land owned by whites. During the planting, tilling, and harvesting of the crops, the white owner provided the funds for seeds, fertilizers, tractors, and other equipment. Labor was provided by the farmer. At the end of the season when the crops were sold, the white owner would be repaid first, and any funds left over would be divided between the tenant farmer and the white owner. For many black farmers, this worked to their extreme disadvantage.

There were no black doctors, dentists, lawyers, or engineers and few black-owned businesses in our community. Most black residents worked at white-owned businesses, on farms, or in white homes as domestic workers.

My father, Walter W. Sullivan Sr., had moved our family from Atlanta to Blakely in 1937, when I was almost four years old, and he established the first black funeral home in Early County. He also operated an ambulance service, where my older brother, Walter Jr., and I helped out. That's how, a year later, in Bainbridge, Georgia, 41 miles south of Blakely, I met the only black physician in southwest Georgia at that time, Dr. Joseph Griffin. It was a life-changing experience for me.

Dr. Griffin had built a 25-bed brick hospital and clinic—an unusual building in that part of the United States at that time, where most structures owned by blacks were made with wooden siding. He was highly admired in the community. He could cure those who were sick or injured, which seemed like magic to me. I already loved science and nature, and I decided that I wanted to be just like Dr. Griffin. I wanted to help people who needed a doctor. And, like Dr. Griffin's patients, my patients would be treated with the respect and dignity they deserved. Black patients would be addressed as "Mrs. Jones" or "Mr. Williams" instead of by their first names, as they were always addressed by white doctors and their staffs.

My quest for equal treatment of patients regardless of race was instilled in me by my father. He had founded the first chapter of the National Association for the Advancement of Colored People (NAACP) in Blakely in the 1930s and brought a lawsuit against the county and state governments because of Georgia's primary voting system, which did not permit blacks to participate. He initiated the annual Emancipation Day celebration in our town, held on January 1, with a parade downtown around the courthouse square and bands, speakers, picnics, and voter recruitment and education programs.

My mother, Lubirda, was a schoolteacher, but because of my father's political activism, she was never able to get a position as a teacher in our local school system during the 20 years my parents lived in Blakely. Instead, she traveled daily to teach in communities outside of Early County, between 14 and 40 miles away. My brother and I were enrolled in the schools where she taught, and we traveled with her.

At age five, after meeting Dr. Griffin, I told my parents that I wanted to become a doctor. "That's wonderful, Louis," they exclaimed. "You would be a great doctor." That was all the confirmation I needed. From that date on, there was never any doubt in my mind that I was going to provide needed medical services in my community with dignity and respect for the patients.

In 1950 I enrolled at Morehouse College. Though my mother was an alumna of Clark College in Atlanta, and my brother had enrolled there a year earlier, I was impressed by the number of black doctors who were alumni of Morehouse, a predominantly black, all-male college.

From Medical School to US Department of Health and Human Services

At Morehouse College, my classmates and I came under the influence of the school's challenging educational and social environment and dedicated faculty and staff, led by the school's president, Dr. Benjamin E. Mays. He was a sophisticated, well-educated man of great integrity and impeccable conduct—a true role model. All of us wanted to be like Dr. Mays. In his eloquent weekly chapel addresses to the students, he challenged us to "reach for the stars and grasp at the moon." He said that each of us was born to make our own unique contribution to the world; our task was to find out what that was and work to achieve it. We were also encouraged to work for the elimination of a segregated society and for the uplifting of ourselves and others.

Four months after graduating from Morehouse in May 1954, I entered Boston University School of Medicine. It was the year of the landmark *Brown v. Board of Education* decision by the US Supreme Court that declared segregation in schools to be unconstitutional. I was the only black in a class of 76 medical students.

My family had only modest resources, but I had no financial concerns about attending medical school. Scholarships were available to financially needy students like me, and medical school tuitions were not in the stratosphere where they are today, costing as much as $60,000 per year. I worked at summer jobs to help cover the costs. The concept of having to borrow and incur massive debt to become a doctor did not exist during my medical school years. When I graduated, I had only $500 in educational debt, which I paid off by the end of my internship year.

After postgraduate training in internal medicine and hematology at New York Hospital–Cornell Medical Center and at Thorndike Laboratory–Harvard Medical Unit at Boston City Hospital, I eventually became a professor of medicine at Boston University and chief of the Division of Hematology at Boston City Hospital.

In 1975, after living 21 years in the northeast, I moved back to Atlanta. Morehouse College had recruited me to be the founding dean of Morehouse School of Medicine, the only predominantly black four-year medical school established in the United States in the twentieth century. After the medical school became independent from Morehouse College on July 1, 1981, I served as president of the medical school until January 20, 1989, when I was appointed by President George H. W. Bush to serve as health and human services secretary.

At that time the Department of Health and Human Services (HHS) had the fourth-largest annual budget in the world: $600 billion, exceeded only by the government budgets of the United States, Japan, and the Soviet Union. (By contrast, the budget of the US Department of Defense was $300 billion in 1989.) HHS had 125,000 employees and managed more than 250 programs, including Social Security, Medicare, Medicaid, the Food and Drug Administration, the National Institutes of Health (NIH), the Centers for Disease Control and Prevention, and many others.

During my tenure as secretary, from 1989 to 1993, HHS achieved much. We launched Healthy People 2000 in September 1990, developed a new food label in 1991, and mounted strong programs to discourage cigarette smoking and other tobacco use. We also persuaded Congress to increase the annual research budget for NIH from $8 billion to more than $13 billion and increased gender and racial diversity among senior leaders at HHS. Our administration saw the appointment of Bernadine Healy, the first female director of the NIH; Antonia Novello, the first female and the first Hispanic surgeon general; Gwendolyn King, the first black female commissioner of the Social Security Administration; and William Toby, the first black administrator of the Health Care Financing Administration (now the Centers for Medicare and Medicaid Services). In 1993, I returned to Morehouse School of Medicine, serving as president until 2002.

As a result of the investment made in me through scholarships available in the 1950s, I was able to make some contributions to society that I otherwise could not have made. Other blacks in my generation could say the same. Mitchell Spellman, for instance, was founding president of Charles Drew School of Medicine in Los Angeles. Augustus White developed the residency program in orthopedic surgery at the Boston Beth Israel Hospital. Asa Yancey was the first black physician to serve as chief medical officer at Grady Hospital in Atlanta. And Claude Organ was the first black chair of surgery at a predominantly white school of medicine, Creighton University.

Today, graduating from medical school with a mere $500 of debt seems unimaginable. With high tuitions for medical school and limited scholarship dollars, it is now common for a medical student to accumulate debts of $150,000 to $250,000 by the time he or she graduates—and some owe even more.

Because of this reality, many college students, especially minority students from low-income families, are discouraged from ever applying to medical school, no matter how much they wish to do so.

According to a 2006 report from the Association of American Medical Colleges (AAMC), the median family income of entering medical students surveyed increased from $50,000 in 1987 to $100,000 in 2006. Even at Morehouse School of Medicine, in 1995 the mean family income of our entering students was $48,500, whereas the mean income for black families nationally at that time was less than $25,000. Our efforts to recruit and graduate students from low-income communities were not as successful as we had hoped they would be.

More recent data from the AAMC show that the median family income for all first-year medical students in the United States was $120,000 in 2014. The median income for black families in the same year was $35,398, according to the Census Bureau. At Morehouse School of Medicine, the median income of first-year medical students (who are mostly minorities) was $76,000 in 2014—less than the median family income for all US medical students but more than twice that of US black families in general.

When minority students give up their dream of becoming a doctor or other health professional, they are depriving themselves, depriving future patients who would benefit from having a more ethnically and racially diverse health care workforce, and depriving the nation of the contributions they could make to improving their lives, their community, and the country.

Another AAMC report, *Altering the Course: Black Males in Medicine*, released in August 2015, found that in 2014 there were 27 fewer black male first-year medical students than there had been in 1978, 36 years earlier—a striking observation.

Could having a minority physician help address the startling health disparities observed between whites and people of color? In 1996, Miriam Komaromy and colleagues documented in the *New England Journal of Medicine* that black and Latino physicians are three to five times more likely than white physicians to establish their offices in the ghetto or barrio, providing services to underserved populations. And a report from the Institute of Medicine in 2003, *Unequal Treatment: Confronting Racial and Ethnic Disparities in Health Care*, documented the conscious and unconscious biases that physicians often have against poor people. Changing the makeup of the health care workforce could change how care is delivered to vulnerable patients.

By allowing our educational system to evolve over the past few decades into one in which so many students in the health professions incur massive debts to support their education, we have also inadvertently created a national environment that has impaired access to health services for too many of our citizens. To more quickly reduce their educational debts, many newly trained health professionals are choosing higher-paying medical specialties instead of primary care for their careers. This has resulted in fewer family physicians, pediatricians, general internists, and psychiatrists than we need.

Developing the Health Workforce the Nation Needs

Given these realities, what can be done to make a career in the health professions more affordable and the health workforce more inclusive? I believe that the nation's health profession schools must work diligently to avoid increasing tuitions further. This will require greater efforts by trustees, presidents, deans, and others in the schools to secure the needed funds from public and private sources to lessen the burden currently placed on health professions students and their families.

To stimulate and support the expansion of health professions education in the nation during the second half of the twentieth century and to avert a predicted shortage of health professionals, Congress enacted a number of bills in the 1960s and 1970s, collectively referred to as "health manpower" legislation. One of the initiatives developed at that time was the National Health Service Corps, which has a program that provides full tuition, covers the cost of books, and pays a living stipend to students who commit to practicing in a federally designated Health Professional Shortage Area for a specified number of years after completion of their postgraduate training. This program has been very effective in supporting future health professionals and placing them in medically underserved rural and urban areas. Unfortunately, it and other scholarship programs were drastically reduced in the 1980s. The American Recovery and Reinvestment Act of 2009 and the Affordable Care Act of 2010 include significant expansion of the National Health Service Corps scholarship program.

Today many health profession students rely extensively on student loan programs to support their years of training. In its August 2015 report, the AAMC stated that among the students graduating from a US medical school in 2014, mean educational debt was $178,000, 31.5 percent of the students had total debt of more than $200,000, and 41.9 percent of black male students had educational debt in excess of $200,000 (the report did not enumerate medical school debt for female students).

A number of novel programs and initiatives have been rolled out recently, aimed at making health profession education more affordable.

The Uniformed Services University of the Health Sciences, for instance, trains health professionals for careers in the military services. Because of their military commitment, the students obtain their education at no cost. Military scholarships are also provided to health profession students in many medical schools in return for their subsequent service as health professionals in the military for a defined period.

The Salina campus of the University of Kansas School of Medicine recruits students committed to becoming primary care physicians and working in medically underserved rural communities in Kansas. Through the medical school's Kansas Bridging Plan, some of the students' educational debts are forgiven in return for practicing in these underserved communities. Several states have similar programs for paying off educational debt, including Louisiana's State Loan Repayment Program, intended to encourage primary care practitioners to serve in Health Professional Shortage Areas, and a Minnesota loan forgiveness program to encourage midlevel providers—physician assistants, nurse practitioners, certified nurse midwives, dental therapists, and others—to practice in rural areas.

Over the years, Morehouse School of Medicine has worked to secure funds for student support from public and private sources. As a result of their commitment to providing primary care and establishing their practices in federally designated medically underserved areas, 19 of the 24 students in the school's first class received National Health Service Corps scholarships.

Policy makers should evaluate these and other strategies for financing health professionals' education to determine whether they represent viable mechanisms for developing the health workforce needed by the nation, removing financial barriers for low- and middle-income students, assisting in the recruitment of physicians to medically underserved communities, and helping increase racial and ethnic diversity in the nation's health professions. Such investments are necessary to ensure that the talents and skills required for our nation's health system will be there in the future.

A fundamental requirement for a strong nation is a healthy population. For the United States, this means having sufficient numbers and sufficient diversity of health professionals in urban and rural communities across the country to promote healthy lifestyles and a culture of wellness, and to care for people who are afflicted by illness or injury. In the US health care system, greater racial and ethnic diversity is essential to providing high-quality care, promoting the cultural competence of health professionals, and developing the trust and confidence in health professionals needed by the people served by the system.

There are no longer separate waiting rooms for white and black patients in Blakely. We've made some progress. But if we do not invest sufficiently today in the education of young health professionals, although we now sit in the same room, we may have a very long wait.

Bridging the Divide between Dental and Medical Care

A cancer patient delays needed dental care before radiation treatment and develops a painful, incurable disease.

Gayathri Subramanian

James sat quietly in our hospital's urgent care dental clinic waiting for preradiation dental triage. He had just been diagnosed with tongue cancer and would soon undergo radiation therapy. Before treatment, he needed all invasive dental treatments completed because

Volume 35, Number 12. December 2016.
Editor's Note: The patient's name in this article has been changed to protect his privacy.

radiation can take an enormous toll on the oral cavity, weakening the teeth and jawbone.

James had been referred to us in 2013 from the radiation oncology department at University Hospital in Newark, New Jersey. Our urgent care dental clinic, also located at University Hospital, is affiliated with the Rutgers School of Dental Medicine, where I'm a faculty member. Hence, I oversee our dental residents as they treat patients who present to the urgent care clinic.

James was unemployed and in his early 50s, with little income and a tough life. He worked odd jobs now and then. He was a smoker—three packs a day for more than 30 years—and a drinker, consuming a few cans of beer a day. His broken-down teeth seemed to bear testimony to years of neglect. He had medical insurance but no dental coverage.

For many of the patients we treat at the urgent care clinic, daily life is such a struggle that brushing and flossing are a low priority. Other patients have never been properly educated about oral hygiene or have little familiarity with the health care system.

James had been aware of a slowly growing mass in his tongue but only sought care when he began having trouble swallowing and started experiencing severe pain that spread to his ear. His smoking and drinking had inevitably contributed to his developing cancer on the floor of his mouth and the base of his tongue. While not a candidate for surgery, he was recommended chemotherapy in conjunction with radiation therapy. Because the treatment would expose his oral structures—including the jawbone, salivary glands, and teeth—to radiation, a dental evaluation was prompted.

A resident examined James's mouth. He was missing several teeth, and his remaining teeth had such advanced decay that conservative management with fillings or root canal treatment would no longer be feasible. He would need nearly 18 tooth extractions. We know that radiation treatment to the jaw can significantly undermine bone healing after teeth are extracted. In about 10 percent of patients who have teeth extracted following radiation (the exact incidence varies), the jawbone is unable to heal adequately and tends to die out, meaning it loses its viable cells and cannot repair or remodel itself anymore. The affected bone (usually in relation to the socket remaining after tooth extraction) loses the protective cover from overlying gum tissue, and because it remains exposed to the mouth, the risk of infections increases. In rare cases, the infections can cause the jaw to weaken and eventually fracture—an often painful disease called osteoradionecrosis, with no known cure. Osteoradionecrosis is known to occur most frequently during the first two years following completion of radiation therapy to the jaw. However, there is a lifelong risk that persists beyond the first two years.

There is no personalized risk-assessment tool to help gauge a patient's risk for developing osteoradionecrosis, although patients who receive more than 50 grays (the unit used to measure radiation dosage) of radiation to the jaw are, in general, at higher risk. It is sometimes difficult to determine whether to recommend saving or extracting questionable teeth, although, in James's case, we knew his situation could only worsen. Leaving him with a mouthful of condemned teeth that would likely deteriorate merely stacked the odds against him.

When I explained all of this to him, however, James declined dental care because he could not afford it. He said his teeth did not hurt him at that time; the debilitating pain he was experiencing was from his tumor, and he just wanted to get through his radiation treatment to ease his pain. We could not deny his decision. Because osteoradionecrosis is rare and poorly predictable, a mandatory dental referral and clearance prior to receiving radiation to the jaw is not yet the standard of care.

Bad News

James completed his course of radiation and chemotherapy at University Hospital, and his subsequent scans showed no evidence of residual disease. He was restricted to a soft pureed diet that could be swallowed a little at a time and had to supplement his minimal intake with a feeding tube in his stomach. Then, nearly a year later, he arrived back at the dental clinic just as we feared, with rampant tooth deterioration and painful abscesses from his infected teeth where the infection had spread beyond the tips of the roots. In several areas, James had yellowish-white pus oozing from his gums from the infection. He was a stoic patient, not prone to showing emotion or complaining. But at this point, he could no longer suffer in silence.

"Doc, the pain is killing me," James moaned while in the dental exam chair. He was ready to get his teeth extracted to relieve the pain.

James told us that he was scheduled to undergo an ear, nose, and throat procedure under general anesthesia within the next week to repair a small skin defect caused by his skin tissue being stretched and thinned postradiation, resulting in a perforation in his cheek. He begged us to perform the extractions at the same time so that he would not be awake for the procedures. Because time was of the essence, we agreed. James now had dental coverage along with his medical insurance, making it possible for him to afford the care he needed. We were able to go into the operating room right after the ear, nose, and throat specialist had repaired the perforation, and we were able to extract all of James's remaining teeth.

For a few months, James seemed to be healing. But in time, a few of his dental extraction sites started to break down, exposing dead bone tissue on both sides of his lower jaw, establishing his diagnosis with osteoradionecrosis. He developed a fungal infection in his mouth—a fallout of an immune system compromised by chemotherapy and radiation treatment. No palliative measures, such as antibiotics, pain medication, antibacterial mouth rinses, or even hyperbaric oxygen therapy, had yet been proven effective, and we knew that James was in danger of losing his jaw to osteoradionecrosis.

In the meantime, James had become dependent on the pain medications he had relied on so heavily to help him through his cancer, its treatment, and now his unremitting pain. As he developed tolerance, the pain medications became increasingly ineffective. For a while, we saw him monthly to monitor his condition, but we couldn't convince him to keep up with these visits, which so rarely seemed to bring him any relief. He comes less these days, maybe once or twice a year, hoping for news of a cure for his disease, but mostly afraid that we might condemn him to having the damaged section of his jaw surgically removed.

Bridging the Artificial Divide

If James had had dental insurance alongside his medical insurance at the time he needed it, his story could have had a very different ending. He could have undergone his 18 tooth extractions well before his radiation treatment, at the same time that an ear, nose, and throat specialist performed his diagnostic biopsy, all under general anesthesia. His extraction sites could have healed by the time his biopsy result was available and his radiation therapy was being planned. Or, even better, James could have taken his oral health seriously enough to have regular health checkups and periodic dental care. His tongue cancer could have been diagnosed several months earlier, and his dentition could have been stable enough to withstand the radiation without the need for extractions.

Instead, by the time James finally obtained dental coverage, the risk of osteoradionecrosis was irreversibly established. By the time he was able to see us monthly, he had developed osteoradionecrosis, and we had nothing substantial to offer him to improve his condition. On the other hand, even if he'd had dental insurance coverage earlier, a plan's annual cap on maximum expenses would likely have left him with significant financial burden.

When oral health is treated as if it were unrelated to overall health—as is the case in this country, where there is "medical" insurance and then there is "dental" insurance—the consequences can be dire. Today, there are more than 108 million people who have no dental insurance, according to the Health Resources and Services Administration. The United States spends more than $64 billion each year on oral health care, out of which only 4 percent is paid for by government programs. According to a 2000 surgeon general's report,

Oral Health in America, for every adult who has no medical insurance, there are three who have no dental insurance, even though it has been estimated that almost everyone experiences dental disease in his or her lifetime.

At the dental school where I teach, many of our patients have low incomes and lack dental insurance. Like James, most would benefit from timely access to oral health care. While dental benefits are required for children under both Medicaid and the Children's Health Insurance Program, dental benefits for adults are optional. Traditional Medicare also does not cover most dental care. Under the Affordable Care Act (ACA), dental coverage for children is now an "essential health benefit." Timely preventive and interventional oral health care for children likely will improve their oral health outcomes and help prevent oral diseases as they age.

However, while the ACA mandates individual health care coverage for all eligible US adults, it does not recognize dental coverage as an essential health benefit for adults, perpetuating the flawed perception of overall health as exclusive and independent of oral health.

The arguments against combining medical and dental benefits, whether valid or otherwise, are primarily financial. Secondarily, they reflect a mind-set that perceives oral health as an optional milestone to strive for.

This artificial divide is especially explicit in a hospital such as ours, which offers urgent oral health care services under the same roof as other health care services. Having traditional insurance allows patients access to health care services elsewhere in the building, but once seated in the dental chair facing a dental emergency, patients often are told that their treatment must be paid for out of pocket.

It has been 16 years since the surgeon general acknowledged the silent epidemic of oral diseases affecting our most vulnerable citizens: poor children, the elderly, and members of racial and ethnic minority groups. Yet poor oral health still disproportionately affects low-income adults, particularly those from racial and ethnic minority groups. It is time that we erased these disparities, particularly for patients with life-threatening illnesses, for whom dental care and medical care are intertwined. Mandating that medical insurance cover essential dental treatments such as tooth extractions, fillings, and root canal procedures, particularly for cancer patients such as James, whose dental health and overall health are so closely related, might be an essential first step. We cannot afford to walk away from our obligation to strive for oral health equity—an integral part of achieving overall health equity—no matter the financial implications.

In Rural Towns, Immigrant Doctors Fill a Critical Need

Immigrant doctors have helped fill physician shortages for years. In the current political climate, are they welcome?

Yasmin Sokkar Harker

Last summer, a headline on Facebook caught my eye. "We Asked Trump Voters 'When Did America Stop Being Great?'" it began. "Their Answers Will Amaze You." The link led to a video of interviews from the America First Unity Rally in Cleveland, Ohio, for which supporters of then presidential candidate Donald Trump had gathered. When did America stop being great? I paused.

At that time, I was still puzzled by the ascendance of Trump as a presidential candidate, and like many other people, I didn't really believe he could win. I would probably have scrolled past the article had it not been for my connection to Cleveland. Cleveland was my birthplace, and although I spent most of my childhood in rural Ohio, I was drawn back to Cleveland for college and then law school.

When did America stop being great? I looked at the grassy lawn that stretched out beside the Cuyahoga River in the video. I looked

Volume 37, Number 1. January 2018.

at the flags, the red caps, and the signs. I clicked play. The first few people responded with vague sentiments: that special-interest groups were "getting their way" and being heard while "the mainstream" was being overlooked, and that Trump was giving "us" (those overlooked individuals) a voice. Then a woman with short brown hair looked directly into the camera and said something unexpected: "I would say about thirty years ago I started noticing . . . I'm in the medical field, and things like . . . all the doctors coming in were coming from foreign countries."

When did America stop being great? When the doctors from foreign countries started coming. When my parents arrived.

I froze. I felt like I had been ambushed. I stopped the video. I replayed it. *Doctors from foreign countries.* I replayed it again, a small wound in my heart slowly expanding.

The Story of My Family

Over the next few months, I sought that video over and over, as if by rewatching it, I could get some answers from this woman. Who was she? She said she was in the medical field—had she worked alongside people like my parents? How did she treat them? Did she know their stories? And why—of all the things she could have chosen to represent when America stopped being great—did she choose physicians?

The story of my family is the story of those *doctors from foreign countries.* I've always thought of it as a wonderful story.

My parents came from their respective countries—my mother from the Philippines and my father from Egypt—to fill a physician shortage that had plagued the United States for decades. They met as residents in a Cleveland hospital in the early 1970s. My mother had been in the country for a few years already and had just purchased her first car, a Mercury Cougar. My father, having just arrived, wanted to learn how to drive. I'm not sure how successful the driving lessons were, but my parents were married shortly afterward. I arrived a year later. When I was three years old, we moved to a small town about 50 miles from Cleveland, where they would both practice for over 30 years.

Our new home was within walking distance of a truck stop on a major interstate. We had several gas stations, car washes, a diner, a McDonald's, and eventually a Wendy's. Behind our house was a wooded area and a creek in which you could sometimes spot turtles and tadpoles. If you continued walking through the woods—past the creek and up a hill—you would emerge into a parking lot behind the Howard Johnson's restaurant and motor lodge. We lived about seven miles from the clinic and the hospital where my parents went to work almost every day for most of my life.

I always wondered: How did I, the child of immigrants from different ends of the globe, grow up where I did? I read about the immigrant enclaves of large cities, about mass immigration to the Chinatowns, the Little Manilas, and Little Indias of Los Angeles, New York, and San Francisco. How did we end up in rural Ohio?

I understand now that the story of my childhood and the story of my life have been shaped by much larger forces: by health care dynamics that brought physicians like my parents to people who badly needed them.

The physicians who cared for the people of my town were almost all immigrants. They were referred to as foreign medical graduates, or FMGs for short. This cadre of FMGs had originated all over the globe: Along with my parents, our town's physicians came from Bulgaria, India, Iran, Jordan, Slovenia, and Taiwan. The on-call schedule that was tacked up on our refrigerator read like a United Nations roll call: Cheng, Syed, Manocher, and so on.

The census data from both 1980 and 1990 show that Ashtabula County, Ohio, in which I spent most of my life, was 95 percent white. For the most part, minorities and immigrants did not have a presence in our rural town. The statistics are consistent with my memories. I don't remember knowing or seeing any people of color or immigrants until much later in my life, with one big exception: my parents and their colleagues.

Many, if not all, of these physicians had left their homes and families behind to build a life far away from everything they knew. I'm sure it was lonely for many of them, but they found friendship in each other. My memories are filled with backyard barbeques and birthday parties. I learned to eat biriyani, rice noodles, and almond jelly alongside hamburgers, potato chips, and ice-cream cake. We were more than statistics about immigrant success: we were creating our lives and writing our own stories.

For decades my parents tended to the people of the town with tenderness and tenacity. Because there weren't many physicians in town, they were in demand. They were tethered to the hospital through telephones and pagers. Our weekend excursions to the mall or the movies were often cut short by the sound of a pager going off. Our phone rang regularly at three or four a.m., and the calls often ended with one of my parents getting dressed and driving off into the night.

For many years my mother worked a 12-hour emergency room shift on Wednesdays. On those days my father would bring my sister and me to the hospital before we went home for dinner. Sometimes my mother would be waiting for us in the on-call room. It was a tiny space located next to the morgue, furnished with a vinyl armchair and narrow bed where the ER doctor could watch television or take a nap while waiting to spring into action. Other times she would be in the emergency room itself, and if I peered past the reception desk, I could see her scurrying to or from a patient's bed, a white coat enveloping her small frame and a stethoscope draped around her neck. I always felt a swell of pride when I saw her like this. I knew that in that moment, she was saving a life.

What I didn't realize at the time was that she also was filling a critical need for physicians in our small, rural town—a need that is just as critical today.

Travel Bans and Patient Care

Like the physicians who worked with my parents 40 years ago, foreign-born physicians today come from a wide array of countries. The top five countries sending physicians to the United States are India, China, the Philippines, Korea, and Pakistan. Across the United States, patients rely on immigrant doctors to prescribe their medications, deliver their babies, perform their surgeries, and ease their pain.

Yet in the current political climate, I worry for those physicians. In January 2017, President Trump signed an executive order barring entry into the United States for the citizens of Iran, Iraq, Libya, Somalia, Sudan, Syria, and Yemen, though the ban met legal opposition. In March, a new executive order barred travel from six predominantly Muslim countries for 90 days. Despite legal challenges, the order went into effect that June. In September, the president unveiled new restrictions on travel to this country, including "enhanced vetting," and in October the Supreme Court dismissed a challenge to the travel ban as moot because of the expiration of the 120-day ban. Though ostensibly meant to make our country safer, these actions have an effect on our nation's health care system as well.

An analysis from the Immigrant Doctors Project found that physicians from the six countries in President Trump's second travel ban provide approximately 2.3 million appointments each year in areas with physician shortages. It also found that 94 percent of Americans live in a community with at least one physician from one of the countries affected by the March travel ban.

Iran and Syria, two of the countries targeted in all three versions of the travel ban, contribute the sixth- and seventh-largest numbers of immigrant physicians in the United States, respectively, with nearly 4,000 physicians having come from Iran and about 3,800 from Syria—according to data from the American Medical Association (AMA).

Many of those physicians work in areas experiencing critical health care shortages, particularly in the Rust Belt (the area of the Midwest that once held thriving coal and steel industries) and Appalachia. It is estimated that today about 10,000 foreign-born doctors work in rural, isolated areas. AMA data suggest that foreign-born doctors are more likely to specialize in primary care—a specialty prone to workforce shortages—and are more likely to serve poor patients on Medicaid. For example, according to statistics from the Alabama Department of Health, in the most medically underserved areas of Alabama, Syrian doctors are the fourth-largest group of foreign-born doctors—behind Indian, Pakistani, and Filipino doctors.

In the months since the travel bans, I have sought such physicians' stories. I read about Suha Abushamma, a Sudanese resident at Cleveland Clinic who, after a trip abroad, returned to the United States only to be turned away; Hooman Parsi, an oncologist scheduled to work in rural California, who remained trapped in Iran amid confusion over the travel ban; and Abdelghani el Rafei, a Syrian medical resident in Minnesota, who could not travel home to see his family. I read stories of confusion, fear, and uncertainty. These physicians' stories could have been like my family's story, but they were cut short before they could truly begin.

In addition to the short-term effects of blocking doctors from entering the United States, the travel bans may be producing a chilling effect, discouraging immigrant physicians from practicing in the US health care system.

For example, as a result of the travel ban, Khaled Almilaji, a Syrian physician, left the United States for Canada. There, he was awarded that country's Meritorious Service Medal for his work with an international relief organization. In another case, the family of Ali Fadhil, an Iraqi doctor who had worked in rural Georgia for several years, started to face harassment in the wake of President Trump's nativist rhetoric. After the travel ban was issued, Dr. Fadhil decided to leave rural America for California, stating that "in the end, this area is just not a place for me to live."

More systematically, some residency programs—such as the one at Einstein Medical Center in North Philadelphia—are now reluctant to match candidates from banned countries, according to reporting by NPR. This reduces the pool of talented young physicians who will come to the United States in the future.

For me, this is a shame. Immigrant doctors have never been a sign that America stopped being great. From the 1970s through the present, they have helped America achieve its greatness.

It is an irony that the areas where immigrant doctors are most needed—the Rust Belt, in particular—are also areas with the strongest support for the president. In the 2016 election, Ashtabula County, my home county, voted 57 percent for Donald Trump, despite having gone for Barack Obama in the two prior elections. My hometown, Geneva Township, went 60 percent for Trump. Of course, there are many reasons why Trump's campaign promises may have appealed to voters there. A floundering economy, lack of opportunities, drug use, and crime are among the problems rural voters from Ashtabula County deal with. But in the context of health care, President Trump's travel bans don't do my hometown any favors.

A Hopeful Sign

Shortly after the first travel ban was signed last January, the AMA sent a letter to the Department of Homeland Security urging officials there not to restrict physicians who have received visas to train, practice, or attend conferences in the United States. In the same letter it affirmed its commitment to students and physicians with Deferred Action for Childhood Arrivals (DACA) status, stating that DACA could introduce 5,400 physicians into our country.

In September the Association of American Medical Colleges (AAMC), joined by 30 other medical associations, filed an amicus brief challenging President Trump's second incarnation of the travel ban. The AAMC argued that the travel ban would exacerbate the nation's health professional workforce shortages, jeopardize progress in medical innovation, and inhibit global research and public health collaborations. The AAMC concluded that the travel ban thus undermines America's ability to avert and respond to health-related national security threats.

Following the third version of the travel ban, the AAMC concluded in a statement that although the revision "eased restrictions" for some health care workers, "they could still face barriers to entry."

I cannot predict what will happen next with our immigration laws. But I do know it behooves our country to oppose nativist and anti-immigrant laws in the future. Indeed, we should support laws—such as the recently introduced Conrad State 30 and Physician Access Reauthorization Act—that encourage immigration and bring immigrant doctors to the regions where they are needed most. The Conrad 30 program allows immigrant doctors to stay in the country in exchange for practicing in underserved areas for at least three years. This bipartisan bill, introduced in April 2017, would renew the program until 2021. The bill has the support of the AMA.

In one hopeful sign, in June the US Citizenship and Immigration Services, a division of the Department of Homeland Security, resumed premium processing of H-1B visas for medical doctors. Such processing for immigrant doctors facilitates the entry of much-needed physicians into our workforce. This is a small step, but a positive one.

My parents are now retired and live near me in New York City. We haven't been back to Ashtabula County for over a decade. The county is still, according to the most recent census, 90 percent white. I am often curious about immigrant families who came after us and about all of those who crossed oceans to settle in the small towns that dot the Rust Belt. What are their lives like today?

The small-town hospital where my parents worked has since been subsumed by a much larger medical conglomerate. But as I scan the physician directory, I see young, smiling faces from medical schools in India, Brazil, and Egypt. I think about them, and I wonder if they plan to stay. I hope so.

An Uninsured Immigrant Delays Needed Care

A physician reflects on the bitter reality of delayed and denied care that her immigrant patient faced more than a decade ago and that many immigrants still face today.

Cheryl Bettigole

In about 2001, long before the Affordable Care Act (ACA) was passed, I took care of a patient I'll never forget. All doctors have them. I was a year and a half out of my family medicine residency, practicing at a safety-net clinic in Philadelphia, Pennsylvania. It was my day to cover the walk-in area of the clinic, where we took care of established patients who were sick and those new to the clinic who couldn't wait the two or three months it took (at the time) for a scheduled appointment. A middle-aged man, soft-spoken and with an anxious look on his face, waited for me in the exam room. He was slightly plump, neatly dressed in a button-down shirt, sweater, and trousers, and he greeted me with great politeness as I entered the room. He was accompanied by one of the clinic's Spanish interpreters, an older woman with a gentle presence and the too-rare ability to explain to us not only our patients' words but also their cultural context.

It was the patient's first visit to our clinic and, in fact, his first visit to any doctor since his arrival in the United States 15 years earlier as a legal immigrant. He sat in a patched vinyl chair facing me, with the interpreter perched near him on the end of the exam table, and explained that he was concerned about a pain in his side and about some weight he had lost without really trying. "But I've been taking a supplement," he told me in Spanish, the interpreter translating in step, "and I think maybe that's what's causing it." He looked up at me hopefully, as if willing me to echo his words.

"How much weight have you lost?" I asked him.

Volume 34, Number 12. December 2015.

"Maybe forty pounds or so," he answered. "But a supplement could do that, couldn't it?"

I began a physical exam. It didn't take long for my fingers to find the grapefruit-size mass in the right side of his abdomen. He winced slightly as I felt around the mass's firm edges. I found it hard to believe that he had failed to notice it himself, and I could see from his guarded expression that he was not surprised by my discovery. I asked him how long it had been there.

"A few months," he said. "Maybe a year, year and a half. I didn't have the money to pay for a doctor."

Like many of the patients I have seen over the years, the man had delayed seeking care in part because he had not yet learned about low-cost safety-net clinics such as ours and assumed that a private physician was his only option. Even if he had known about us earlier, our clinic had a waiting time of several months for new patients and could hardly keep up with the existing demand for its services.

"I Didn't Want to Spend Everything I Had"

Our clinic had a contracted referral system that allowed us to obtain necessary imaging studies for uninsured patients without charging them; with approval from our clinical director, the clinic could cover the cost of the studies at our local hospital. We were fortunate, and rare, in this regard. With the interpreter's help, I explained to my patient that I wanted him to have an ultrasound done to help me understand what the mass was, and then I gave him a referral for the study to be done at the hospital's radiology department, which would send me the report.

As I sent him out, I hoped I was wrong about his diagnosis. There are benign abdominal masses but few that cause weight loss such as he had described. About a week later, I received the results of my patient's ultrasound: they indicated stage IV renal cell carcinoma, a type of very advanced kidney cancer. I called my patient and arranged for him to see a nephrologist at a local hospital, who sent me a report a few days after the visit. The nephrologist confirmed that the tumor was inoperable. His report ended simply, "Advised comfort measures."

With a feeling of dread, I asked my patient to come see me to discuss the report. We talked about his diagnosis and about what it meant to him. He spoke with his shoulders bowed and his words coming slowly. "I run my own business. I've worked hard and saved what I could to build a life here for my family, for my two daughters. When I first noticed the pain, I thought about seeing a doctor, but doctors are expensive. I didn't want to spend everything I had worked for on doctor and hospital bills."

Stage IV renal cell carcinoma is a diagnosis I've never seen before or since. Although there is no routine screening test for renal cell carcinoma, the majority of patients are diagnosed at earlier stages, and the prognosis is dramatically different depending on the stage at diagnosis. For those diagnosed at stage I (in which tumors are often found incidentally because of an imaging scan done for another reason), five-year survival is more than 80 percent. The survival rate drops to 74 percent at stage II, in which tumors have grown to more than seven centimeters but remain confined to the kidney. The survival rate falls to 53 percent at stage III (the cancer has spread locally) and then plummets to 8 percent at stage IV (there is distant metastasis). Had my patient sought care when he first noticed symptoms instead of waiting for months, he would have had a chance at surviving.

As it was, since the specialist had made it clear there were no effective curative treatment options to offer, I set about trying to make my patient's last few months as comfortable as possible. Ordinarily, I would have referred him to one of the many high-quality hospice programs available in Philadelphia. A program such as that could have monitored his need for pain medication, helped with any home care requirements, and offered emotional support for his family. But my patient was uninsured, and my multiple phone calls failed to find a hospice provider that would accept an uninsured patient.

The Best We Could Do

"I'd like to refer a patient," I said to each of the cheerful voices that answered my calls. "But . . . he has no insurance. Can you accept him?" I mentioned that we were trying to get him covered under Medicaid. Some simply said no; others suggested different hospice programs that they thought might accept an uninsured patient (although they never did); and most suggested that I call back once my patient had insurance. When I tried to help him obtain Medicaid coverage, we hit roadblocks there as well. I filled out the application for him, and he took it to the welfare office, with "metastatic renal carcinoma" written in capital letters across the top to make sure it couldn't be missed. But he was told that his savings put him over the financial threshold for Medicaid and that he was too young to qualify for Medicare. I learned years later that there were programs under which he might have qualified for Medicaid, but the caseworker didn't mention any other options. Given gaps in training, the caseworker might not have known that they existed any more than I did at the time.

In the end, all I could offer was medication for his pain, a service that hospice would ordinarily have provided, and my support to him and to his family. A few months after his first visit to my clinic, at what turned out to be his last visit in the office, I gave his daughter my pager number so that she could call if his pain medication stopped working. I still remember standing in my living room one night a few days before he died, phone held in one hand, using the other to page through reference books to find instructions on how to adjust the dose of morphine for cancer pain. At the same time, I couldn't help but wonder how this could possibly be the best I could do for my patient, considering the wealth of health care resources my city has to offer. If my patient had had insurance, a trained hospice team and palliative care expert could have done far more to ease his final days than I could manage with my lack of experience or specialized training.

After my patient's death, his daughter called and thanked me profusely for my efforts, but I was painfully aware of all the ways in which I, along with our health care system, had failed him. Her gratitude made me feel like a fraud, too aware of what would have been different if I had known more, both about end-of-life care and about how to advocate within the convoluted world of Medicaid eligibility.

Immigrant Care

In the years that have passed since my patient's death, I've come to better understand why so many of my immigrant patients come into the health care system too late to get the help that they need. The central fact that immigrants to this country know about our health system, if they know nothing else, is that it is hugely expensive for those without health insurance. Prior to the ACA, small businessmen such as my patient often couldn't afford to buy their own coverage. Many of my other immigrant patients work in service industries that rarely provide insurance to their employees. With the advent of the ACA, many who couldn't previously afford insurance can purchase coverage in the exchanges or (in some states) may qualify for Medicaid. Yet millions of undocumented workers remain barred from these programs, and many have no way of becoming insured. What's more, millions of legal immigrants are barred from Medicaid until they have been residents for five years. During this gap period, they may suffer serious medical problems and, despite their legal status, lack access to care. State laws make exceptions for some immigrants, such as pregnant women and children, but the rules vary from state to state.

In its series "Paying Till It Hurts," the *New York Times* has done much to publicize the fact that our health care system charges the uninsured much more than those with coverage, garnishing wages and working out payment arrangements that can last for years and can tip struggling families into poverty. As other groups have gained coverage through the ACA, immigrants and their children make up an increasing and disproportionate percentage of those who remain uninsured and at risk from these extraordinarily high charges, according to economist Eric Seiber, among other scholars. Word travels quickly in immigrant communities, and my patients are well aware of this risk.

It is true that the ACA has brought real benefits to immigrants, increasing the number of people able to obtain insurance, both via the exchanges and, in participating states, via the Medicaid expansion. But in the end, I fear that many immigrants, both those here legally and those who are undocumented, may still die the same early, painful deaths our health system could not prevent more than 10 years ago.

In 15 years working at safety-net clinics with large immigrant populations from all over the world, both before and after the ACA, I have too often heard similar stories of care that was delayed or denied to uninsured immigrant patients: The woman who felt a lump in her breast and ignored it as it grew month after month, until finally her sister-in-law found out and brought her to the clinic. She was diagnosed with stage III breast cancer at age 35. Or the young woman who broke her ankle and waited four months in exquisite pain before finally finding her way to our doors. The man whose hypertension was diagnosed only after his kidneys failed because he lacked access to basic health care that would have identified his condition sooner. Or the paraplegic man who managed on his own for decades without medical care, using an ancient wheelchair and dressing his decubitus ulcers with the help of family members, until a pressure sore that went all the way down to the bone of his sacrum finally led him to our clinic.

These stories should not come from a major US city that is home to some of the finest health care institutions in the country. They should not happen in a civilized society. But they did. Many of these patients would have been eligible for "emergency Medicaid," which covers treatment for life-threatening conditions for noncitizens and legal immigrants who are subject to the five-year bar. But through a combination of language and literacy barriers, lack of familiarity with the US health care system, the administrative complexity of the application system, and long waiting times for appointments at safety-net clinics, they remained uninsured and without care.

Over the years my colleagues and I have learned how to navigate these systems for our patients, when and how to ask for help, and who to call for urgent cases. I've learned who to call when, as happens so often, my seemingly eligible patients are denied coverage through a Byzantine bureaucratic process. Often, they're not actually told no, but their application is repeatedly lost or labeled as incomplete, and their phone calls go unreturned by overwhelmed caseworkers who sometimes lack the training to understand immigrants' complex situations.

With this knowledge, built up over more than a decade, I can often get critical help to individual patients. Other times, however, it is too late. I am troubled that we continue to allow labyrinthine systems of health care access for vulnerable patients to deny them the help they need and for which they are eligible.

A Hot-Button Issue

In the early days of the debates around what became the ACA, a colleague asked if I would be willing to testify about the need for affordable health insurance in our state. My patient with renal cell carcinoma was one of the reasons I said yes. There is something truly bitter about a dying patient who cannot even access hospice care. The patients who came into my care too late have inspired me to join with many colleagues to write and speak out for expanded access to care and to dispel the mistaken notion that all physicians opposed the law. Given the political atmosphere of the time, the president and many legislators made a calculated decision not to propose universal access, nor to touch the "hot-button issue" of health care coverage for immigrants. The law that passed was a vast improvement on the health care status quo, but many immigrants were left out.

One-quarter of US children have at least one immigrant parent, and almost all of these children are citizens. These children and others who live in mixed-status families (that is, families in which one or more members are undocumented) are at particularly high risk of remaining uninsured. The ACA increases funding for community health centers such as the ones I have worked in, helping to improve access to primary care for many communities. But safety-net clinics are designed to provide primary care and lack the infrastructure and resources to provide more complex care, such as chemotherapy, surgery, fracture care, or hospice services. The costs of chemotherapy alone often run into the tens of thousands of dollars—far beyond the range of these clinics or the average patient without health insurance. Community health centers and safety-net hospitals are essential for immigrant patients, but they are no substitute for health insurance coverage. The belief that these patients can get the care they need through an emergency department or other safety-net institution, which rarely offer cancer treatment or nonemergency surgery to those without health insurance, is simply not true.

According to the Urban Institute, many immigrants do not understand the rules of Medicaid eligibility and fear possible deportation of undocumented family members if they apply. The eligibility rules are complex: they depend on the details of an individual's immigration status, duration of residence in the country, age, sex, health status, and income, and they vary from state to state. Immigrants with limited English proficiency need additional assistance with the process and are at particular risk of remaining uninsured even when eligible. Other challenges include rising caseloads among workers who process the applications, complex applications, and requests for obscure and hard-to-find information such as the Social Security numbers of applicants' parents (even though this is not actually required). And even if they do finally get covered, beneficiaries are typically required to recertify every 6 to 12 months. These factors lead to substantially lower enrollment in Medicaid among eligible immigrants than the US population as a whole, researchers have found.

Linkages to community-based organizations, including those that provide free legal assistance and access to people who can act as trusted navigators and information sources, can make a real difference for immigrant communities. Ultimately, however, we need to offer affordable coverage options to all immigrants and to communicate effectively with these communities about how to obtain the coverage they need.

An Impossible Choice

In 2001, after my patient's death from renal cell carcinoma, I feared that our health care system was creating an economic trap for immigrants in which they could work their whole lives to build financial security for their families only to face a choice between turning every cent over to the health care system or dying an early, preventable death. Now, in 2015, having worked like so many others to create a better system with improved access to decent-quality, affordable care, I am all too aware that not enough has changed for my immigrant patients. Too many remain systematically excluded from access to the health care they need. And the soaring costs of health care for the uninsured still make it all too likely that the next time an immigrant patient feels a mass in his belly and worries, he will think about seeing a doctor and, with a heavy sigh, decide to wait.

6

Aging and End-of-Life Care

"I Don't Want Jenny to Think I'm Abandoning Her"

Views on Overtreatment

A palliative care physician helps a cancer patient cope with her coming death, while her oncologist struggles to give up treatment.

Diane E. Meier

In between seeing patients with the palliative care team at Mount Sinai Medical Center in New York City, I received from my secretary a message from someone seeking an office palliative care consultation. The patient, whom I'll call Jenny, wanted to talk to me before she made an appointment, so I called her late in the day after the rest of the team had gone home. Jenny's voice was upbeat and cheerful as she told me how she had found me—from an internet search—and why she had called. She was in her late 50s, a practicing clinical psychologist with a husband and a daughter recently graduated from college. She had been diagnosed with stage IV non-small-cell lung cancer six years earlier.

When I heard this I wrinkled my brow. Nobody lives six years with this kind of cancer, I thought to myself. Something's odd here. Jenny wanted to see me to make sure her medical team was paying attention to what mattered most to her: her quality of life. There was nothing urgent; she was in no pain. We agreed to meet a couple of weeks later.

She came into the office with her husband, looking totally out of place amidst the frail geriatric population that we generally see in our practice. Elegant, slender, with a gorgeous head of curly blonde hair, Jenny was nothing like what I had expected. Her cancer story, too, was atypical.

She was diagnosed with cancer after experiencing a persistent cough. By the time she had a surgical removal of the tumor, the dis-

Volume 33, Number 5. May 2014.
Editor's Note: The pseudonym "Jenny" was used to protect the privacy of the patient and her family. "Jenny's" oncologist was not named for privacy reasons as well.

ease had already spread outside the lung. She then began chemotherapy and radiation at a major New York City cancer center. She became attached and grateful to the oncologist managing her treatment. Over six years she'd seen periods of remission during which she and her husband traveled the world while maintaining her busy clinical psychology practice and raising their daughter. With each recurrence or progression of disease, her oncologist thought of a new approach to try, and each one worked. Her disease was stable, and her quality of life was good. She hoped she might turn this cancer into a chronic disease instead of a death sentence.

What-Ifs

Given how well Jenny appeared to be doing, I wondered why she was in my office. Jenny described herself to me as a "control freak"—someone who needed to know what to expect and what might happen to her. "Better to know and plan for the worst," she told me. "That way I don't have to worry about it." Over the years she realized that her oncologist was unwilling—in her view, unable—to talk to her about the what-ifs of her cancer. What if this next treatment doesn't work? What if my disease progresses and I can no longer function the way I want to? What will that be like? Will I be in pain? Will I suffocate? How will my husband and daughter take care of me? Where and how will I die? What will I need? Healthy and happy as Jenny appeared, the uncertainty and the unknown were consuming her.

Her oncologist's reaction to each setback was to redouble his efforts to get the cancer under control. Her what-ifs were met with, "We don't have to worry about that."

As a psychologist, Jenny eventually reasoned that her oncologist was unable to face the possibility—indeed, probability—that Jenny would die of this disease. So Jenny came to me, hoping I could give her some answers.

We talked about possibilities. Given the unusual course of her cancer to date, I admitted the real possibility that her oncologist could continue to find ways to keep it at bay. I explained that I could become a part of her treatment team to focus on her quality of life, provide the straight answers she sought, and participate in her desire to plan for the worst while continuing to hope for the best. She relaxed and smiled, expressing relief that her concerns had been validated and that a means of addressing them was in sight.

We talked about what she might expect as her lung cancer progressed, including increased fatigue and weakness, pain, and shortness of breath, and exactly how we could manage these. She wanted to know what it was like to die.

The natural dying process for a cancer patient—for any patient, for that matter—usually involves progressive fatigue, more and more time in bed or chair, more and more sleepiness, progressing to coma and a peaceful death. We talked about what the moment of death was like: slower and slower breathing, with pauses in between breaths, and during one of those pauses, she would die. She asked what would happen if she had pain and symptoms that couldn't be controlled. I explained that virtually all symptoms were manageable with palliative care. If necessary, there was the option of sedation, but it was quite unusual to need that. She followed my words closely and nodded her head, seeming relieved that she need not fear terrible suffering in her final days.

We talked about hospice and what it provides, which would include services such as a team available to come to her home 24/7, as well as equipment, medicine, and training and support for her husband and daughter. If things ever got too difficult at home, she could go to an inpatient hospice setting with around-the-clock nursing and medical care.

Toward the end of our conversation, Jenny said she was worried that her oncologist would feel upset or hurt because she came to see me and that he might not be comfortable working with me on her care. I was worried about that, too. I offered to call him. I would make no treatment recommendations for her without talking to him first.

The relief on the couple's faces was palpable. Something huge and terrifying—and, to Jenny's oncologist, unspeakable—had been brought within her compass. Smiling and excited, Jenny shifted the conversation to talk about her book groups and what she was reading and writing. They left the office with a follow-up appointment three months out.

With some trepidation, I called her oncologist and explained everything. To my relief, and that of Jenny and her husband, he agreed to work together with me on Jenny's care.

The Disease Progresses

For the following 18 months, Jenny received care from both her oncologist and me. We remained in regular email and telephone contact. When she learned, several months after we first met, that her disease had progressed, the oncologist tried another experimental treatment to which Jenny responded well.

For another year, things remained stable, until Jenny began to feel increasingly tired and started to have difficulty focusing her attention and memory. Because of the memory lapses, she worried that she should no longer continue her psychotherapy practice. With her oncologist's agreement, we tried corticosteroids to reduce the swelling around the tumors in her brain and psychostimulants to improve energy and mood, which helped. She kept practicing but canceled a major trip and conserved her energy for home and work. She had no pain and experienced some shortness of breath but only when she ran for the bus or climbed a flight of stairs.

Several months after she first noticed the memory problems, she awoke with a headache and blurred vision. Brain imaging showed an enlarging mass that was progressing despite systemic chemotherapy and corticosteroids.

Jenny came to see me in the office to talk about this new reality. Her oncologist was recommending intrathecal chemotherapy, a treatment that involves placing a reservoir inside the brain in order to administer chemotherapy directly into the site where the tumor mass sits, in the hope of shrinking it. Jenny wanted my opinion on whether she should accept this therapy, but I was unfamiliar with the data on the procedure. I told her I would ask her oncologist about it, and we'd get back to her.

I called him, and after an exchange of pleasantries, I got down to the matter at hand. "Jenny was in today, and she mentioned that you had suggested intrathecal chemo for her brain metastases," I said. "I told her I'd call to find out what you anticipated from this approach, since this is outside my expertise. What are you hoping we can accomplish with this treatment?"

After a brief pause, he spoke. "It won't help her."

I struggled for a response. "Would you want me to encourage her to go ahead with it anyway?" I asked, finally.

After another pause, this one longer and more awkward than the last, he said, "I don't want Jenny to think I'm abandoning her."

A New Perspective

His comment struck me. For years I had tried and failed to understand why so many of my physician colleagues persisted in ordering tests, procedures, and treatments that seemed to provide no benefit to patients and even risked harming them. I didn't buy the popular and cynical explanation: physicians do this for the money. It fails to acknowledge the care and commitment that these same physicians demonstrate toward their patients. Besides, Jenny's oncologist would make no money from the intrathecal chemotherapy procedure. Instead, the impulse motivating him to order more tests and interventions was as an expression of his continued commitment to helping her.

It seemed that the only way Jenny's oncologist knew to express his care and commitment for her was to order tests and interventions. He felt that to stop doing this was akin to abandoning her. His words transformed my understanding of what I've viewed as inexplicable behavior in the face of progressive and terminal illness.

It was ironic as well. The only way in which Jenny felt her oncologist had actually abandoned her, as she told me, was by his unwillingness to talk with her about what would happen when treatment stopped working.

How did Jenny and her oncologist come to see things so differently? Patients and families, especially those dealing with a progressive cancer, know that every life ends in death. They assume their doctors are trained and knowledgeable about end of life as well, and they assume that if the doctor recommends more tests and treatments, he thinks they will help in some way. Patients and families also assume that doctors will tell them when time is running out, what to expect, and how best to navigate these unknown and frightening waters.

But many doctors don't do these things. Most are, in fact, completely untrained in these aspects of the human experience. Medical school and residency have traditionally provided little or no training on how to continue to care for patients when disease-modifying treatments no longer work. Physicians are trained to make diagnoses and to treat disease. Untrained in skills such as pain and symptom management, expert communication about what to expect in the future, and achievable goals for care, physicians do what we have been trained to do: order more tests, more procedures, more treatments, even when these things no longer help. Even when they no longer make sense.

Training Physicians

So how do we fix this? Most policies to change physicians' behaviors have focused on restructuring financial incentives. If we pay more (or less), the theory goes, for certain activities, physicians' behaviors will change. The evidence correlating financial incentives and physicians' behavior changes is mixed at best, however, and it is too early to judge their impact on patient care quality and costs.

Policies aimed at fundamental change in physicians' behaviors will require more than financial incentives. Doctors care deeply about their patients, and most aim to express that care exactly as they were taught to express it. To change behavior, we must change the education and training of young physicians and the professional and clinical culture in which they practice. New doctors should learn about the management of symptoms such as pain, shortness of breath, fatigue, and depression, with intensive training on doctor-patient communication: how to relay bad news, how to stand with patients and their families until death, and how to help patients and families make the best use of their remaining time together. Armed with different training, Jenny's oncologist might have been able to express his care and commitment in ways that better suited his patient's needs.

The Affordable Care Act contains no provisions aimed at standardizing and overhauling undergraduate and graduate medical education. Graduate medical education (GME) funding from the Medicare trust funds is the main source of financial support for physician training after medical school. At least in theory, policy makers could tie such support to training priorities important to Medicare beneficiaries, such as basic palliative care skills and knowledge.

At present, however, government has few levers to use in influencing the content and quality of physician training. A 2010 report from the Medicare Payment Advisory Commission suggested linking Centers for Medicare and Medicaid Services support for GME funding to the achievement of medical competencies and standards aligned with payment for quality outcomes. Subsequently, a joint initiative by the Accreditation Council for Graduate Medical Education and the American Board of Internal Medicine developed 22 training milestones (knowledge, skills, attitudes) to ensure certain competencies for internal medicine residents, such as effective communication with patients and caregivers.

Today, virtually 100 percent of medical school–affiliated teaching hospitals have palliative care teams. Recent data show that the younger the physician, the higher his or her familiarity and comfort with palliative care. Resources for teaching these skills are widely available and could be standardized and scaled to reach all trainees. A working group of the American Academy of Hospice and Palliative Medicine is developing a set of competencies, milestones, and certain essential tasks physicians should know, called "Entrustable Professional Activities," in palliative medicine for medical residents.

Saying Good-bye

As we talked, Jenny's oncologist had a change of mind about his treatment recommendation. "We're not going to do that," he told me. He called Jenny and told her that he didn't think intrathecal chemotherapy would help her and that he thought it was time to involve hospice. Jenny gave up working, entered a hospice program, and settled in at home. There, her husband and daughter, along with the hospice team and I, took care of her.

Toward the end of her life, Jenny told me she wanted to thank her oncologist and say good bye. Once she began receiving home hospice care, he had neither called nor visited. Her feelings of gratitude and connection to him had only grown as she prepared to die. With her permission, I called him.

"Jenny asked me to call you because she would love to see you," I said.

"Isn't she at home on hospice?" he said. "There's nothing I can do for her now."

Though he sounded slightly irritated by my call, I thought about how many such losses he had experienced in his oncology practice and how painful and distressing the prospect of Jenny's death might feel to him. I persisted.

"She feels very attached and grateful to you," I said. "She wants to thank you, and she wants to say good-bye. It would be great if you could stop by."

He had not visited a patient at home before, but he agreed to go. She thanked him for his amazing care and for giving her so many good years after her lung cancer was diagnosed. After that visit, she lived only a few more days.

I am grateful to Jenny's oncologist for reminding me that the commitment to care and help is behind physicians' recommendations to their patients—recommendations firmly based on what they learned during their training. Both Jenny and her oncologist wanted to sustain their human connection, the relationship between doctor and patient that is at the heart of quality of care. With the right training and skills, doctors can honor that relationship throughout their patient's experience of illness, even and especially when disease-focused treatment is no longer beneficial. Our patients, and their doctors, deserve no less.

The Fall

Aligning the Best Care with Standards of Care at the End of Life

When her mother is hurt, a health care executive finds that the standardized care she championed isn't always appropriate.

Patricia Gabow

As the former CEO of Denver Health, a large safety-net health care system in Colorado, where I also served as chief medical officer for most of my 20-year tenure as CEO, I was a vigorous proponent of using the best available data to create standards of care. I embraced this as an essential pathway to reduce care variation and improve quality. Since a majority of our patients were members of minority communities, creating evidence-based standard care pathways for every person also seemed a way to reduce disparity.

Clearly, I was a believer in a standardized approach to care. But when my 94-year-old mother sustained a fall, my strong commitment to standards waned.

Volume 34, Number 5. May 2015.

The Need for Standards of Care

The belief in standards of care led Denver Health to an array of interventions to reduce care variation and improve quality. The first foray into this territory was almost two decades ago with the development of "clinical pathways," or guided approaches for common medical problems. As many readers will remember, this approach was greeted by cries of "cookbook medicine," reflecting, in part, physicians' long history of autonomy and their belief that they always tried to do what was best for the patient. Without care standards, however, we see variability in the care of patients with similar clinical problems—and some of that care is suboptimal. Therefore, my response to the criticism was: "Better a cookbook recipe that worked than a *trial-and-error* approach that failed."

Denver Health became an early adopter of computerized provider order entry with standard order sets for an array of conditions. For example, instead of relying on each doctor to remember best practices, a standard order set was created for diabetic ketoacidosis, an acute diabetic complication. This reduced patient time in the intensive care unit (ICU) and the hospital, and it reduced acute treatment complications.

Then, in 2005, Denver Health began implementing "Lean" principles and processes, built on the Japanese automaker Toyota's focus on respect for people and continuous improvement to reduce waste and improve quality. We used Lean's "Rapid Improvement Event" process to create standard approaches to care for interventions such as anticoagulation after surgery, to reduce the occurrence of postoperative deep venous thrombosis. These efforts and other similar interventions produced improved quality of care, with outcomes such as achieving blood pressure control in 70 percent of patients compared to a national average of about 50 percent and an observed-to-expected hospital mortality ratio of less than one, saving many lives.

We need standards of care. But when I found myself confronting an array of standards in the emergency department with my mother,

I began to see that we need to adapt standards for the patient population and the individual patient being treated.

About My Mother

My mother, Terese, was the daughter of an immigrant father who sent his two sons and my mother to college during the Depression, enabling all of them to become schoolteachers. My mother's first husband (my father) was killed in World War II, and she remarried a fellow teacher a decade later. They spent many years teaching in rural Pennsylvania, where they were beloved by generations of students. Last Christmas my mother received 150 cards, some from students she had taught 60 years ago, reflecting on the difference she had made in their lives.

About 15 years ago my mother began to develop dementia. My stepfather was a devoted caregiver, allowing them to live independently on their tree-filled acre of land in St. Petersburg, Pennsylvania. When he died suddenly almost five years ago, it was not feasible for my mother to live alone, 2,000 miles from me, her only child. So we moved her to Denver. Given the extent of her memory loss and her tendency to wander, she needed to live in a dedicated memory unit that provided for the special needs of dementia patients with the presence of 24-hour caregivers. After an initial bumpy adjustment to my stepfather's death and the move, she settled in well. The caregivers and even family members of other residents loved her. She told everyone she loved them, hugged them, and labeled most of them the "teacher's pet," continuing to manifest the true generosity of spirit that made her so beloved by her students and earned her the nickname of "Mother Teresa."

Over the ensuing five years her dementia slowly worsened, and by the late summer of 2014 her conversation frequently became a "word salad." She started eating less, often slept in a chair in the memory unit's living room, and was less steady on her feet. My mother remained happy and kind but could no longer follow commands or understand the reason for anything uncomfortable, including the simplest procedures. Even a blood pressure measurement caused dismay.

My mother and I continued our weekly ritual of going to Saturday evening church service followed by dinner. On the night of Saturday, August 29, 2014, after services and dinner, I was getting ready to drive her to her home. We walked out of my front door and down the one step to the patio. Thinking my mother was stable, I turned to lock the door. The next sound I heard was the crack of her head hitting the flagstone, and my next vision was of her sprawled out on the patio—a sound and sight locked in my mind forever.

She did not lose consciousness and had no obvious broken bones, but she had a large cut on her arm, a small cut above her eye, a rapidly developing black-and-blue mark on her head, and a black eye. I called out to my husband, who was in the house, and we tried to get her up. But even with her small frame and my husband's weight-lifting prowess, we could not. So her encounter with a health system's standards of care began.

Going against the Grain

Having been at Denver Health for 40 years, including my two decades as CEO, I knew almost all the physicians and many of the other employees. I called Denver Health's emergency services director, asking if an ambulance could take my mother to her residence. I was hoping to bypass the standard for the ambulances to deliver patients only to a hospital emergency department (ED), which I thought would be a strange and troubling place for her. As I could not assess her injury, he strongly recommended we bring her to the ED, which we reluctantly did.

The paramedics arrived promptly and, following standard procedure for a head trauma, wanted to put her in a collar. I knew she wouldn't tolerate that and asked them not to do it. Instead, they expertly loaded her onto the stretcher with a scoop, keeping her head stable. Arriving at the ED, we were taken into a trauma room and greeted by the nurse and attending physician. I explained my mother's condition and her inability to tolerate even the simplest intervention. I knew my mother well. Given her strong religious belief in a heavenly home and previous conversations with her and my stepfather regarding end-of-life care, I told her health care team that her goals were comfort and peace, and a prompt return to familiar surroundings. I asked that they not place an intravenous line, which would be used for fluid or medication administration if needed, or to draw blood for laboratory tests. Then, after the initial monitor readings, I asked that they turn the monitor off, since no reading or alarm was supposed to elicit a response, given that she was a "do not resuscitate" patient.

Although my requests did not comply with the standard approach for a patient who has sustained a fall and was brought to the ED by ambulance, the team understood my concerns and agreed that a nonstandard approach was appropriate. Given her head trauma, the next standard step would have been to perform a computed tomography (CT) scan. This would have been yet another unnecessary step, as there would be no finding that would lead to my agreeing to a neurosurgical procedure on my elderly mother. Again, the team agreed to deviate from the standard.

By this time, my mother said her wrist hurt. The attending recommended obtaining wrist X-rays, revealing three nondisplaced breaks, and the orthopedic service team was called. The ED attending turned her attention to the large laceration on my mother's forearm. She said it would be easier to care for and more comfortable for my mother if it was sutured. This seemed reasonable, and the physician proceeded to inject the wound with a local anesthetic using a small needle. "Ouch," my mom cried out. "Why are you doing that?" She asked her to stop. But the local anesthetic quickly took effect, and the attending was able to close the wound with eleven sutures and no further discomfort to my mother. The orthopedic service recommended a plaster splint for her arm rather than surgery, a standard of care that I could accept.

A Tough Decision

By 12:30 a.m. on Sunday morning, about four hours after entering the ED, we were ready to go home—almost. Although my mother was not complaining of any pain in her pelvis, hips, or legs, the ED attending said that the standard of care would be to get her out of bed and see her walk. But my mother was exhausted by now, and I asked that the attending not get her up. She reluctantly agreed. In retrospect, I should have accepted this standard. Back at her residence, my mother would not put weight on her right leg and was complaining of hip pain when she moved.

This resulted in another trip to the ED and a right hip X-ray, which revealed a classic hip fracture (so-called "valgus-impacted femoral neck fracture" in orthopedic terminology). I was entering more difficult terrain in my efforts to honor her goals for care. The orthopedic service explained that the standard of care for this injury was a surgical procedure that would fix the fracture by pinning the hip with three screws.

On the one hand, I felt uncomfortable and a little anxious about potentially denying her appropriate care, especially since she fell when she was on my watch. On the other hand, I did not believe this standard of care was ideal for a 94-year-old with severe dementia. I tried to visualize the first postoperative day in the ICU for her, the strange surroundings filled with constant activity, so unlike the quiet environment of her memory unit. I pictured the intravenous line, which she would try to take out, leading to soft restraints that she would also struggle to get out of. Then sedation and a downward spiral. Every part of this would seem like torture to her—and I would have to watch this torture. Given her lack of physical activity and the fracture's stability, any other option, even including a wheelchair, would seem more acceptable for her.

I asked the resident to imagine the ICU stay, too, and how it was misaligned with our goals for comfort and peace. I wanted to take my mother back to her home. Yet this was too radical a deviation from the standard of care for the resident's comfort. The chief of orthopedics was out of town, but I called him up. I knew him well, had great respect for him, and he had recently operated on my healthier 89-year-old mother-in-law's broken hip with a great outcome. I explained my desire to avoid surgery in my mother's circumstance. The chief of orthopedics had trained in Europe, where the standards of care would include nonoperative management of this stable, nondisplaced fracture in someone with dementia and her age, and he and the team agreed to the approach.

We went home with only Tylenol for pain, the goal of starting physical therapy in several days, and a simple Velcro-attached plastic splint for her arm. Somehow, although none of us could figure it out, she had managed to remove the previous plaster splint—no doubt a whole night's work for her.

Within a week, my mother was walking 30 feet with the help of a physical therapist. The therapist even had her pedaling a stationary bike—quite surprising since my mother had never ridden a bike in her life. She had no pain. Her primary care doctor's physician assistant removed her stitches, and follow-up X-rays were taken at her residence, revealing that the wrist and hip fractures were stable. Her orthopedic surgeon released her from his care with no restrictions or additional X-rays needed.

The Bigger Picture

While the motivation for my decisions was my mother's comfort, the decisions had significant cost implications for Medicare and her supplemental insurance. At a minimum, the total charge for the likely surgical procedure, an expected three-day stay in the ICU, and several other days in the hospital would have been approximately $156,000. While the amount paid to the hospital would be considerably less than the charges, the cost would still be substantial. Additionally, there may have been a costly stay in a rehabilitation facility. More importantly, these expenditures would have been of no value to my mother and, in fact, would have reduced the quality of the remaining days of her life.

The physical and mental downward course for my mother that had begun several months before the fall continued, and a month after the fall, we enrolled her in home hospice at her residence, providing additional care and equipment, such as a hospital bed. By October 21, she did not want to get out of bed, and by October 24, it was clear her earthly days were numbered. She died on Sunday, October 26, in her sunny, plant-filled little apartment room in the memory unit, with my husband and me holding her hand, her iPod headphones in her ears, listening to Perry Como sing "Ave Maria," her favorite song.

To my mind, deviating from the standard approaches to care was clearly the best care for my mother. It gave her two more months of a calm and happy life and a peaceful death. I still believe in standards of care. For many patients, they provide protection from unwarranted and possibly deleterious variation. But my perspective has shifted a bit. Now I ask myself different questions. Could we adapt standards of care, particularly at the end of life, to be more flexible? Could there be branch points reflecting a patient's age, overall condition, and most of all their desires and true best interest?

I also wonder, was it possible for me to deviate from the standards of care, opting for a less invasive approach, only because I had been the CEO of the health system? I was a physician who knew the caregivers, and none of the physicians at Denver Health were getting paid more to do more. Was it possible to avoid surgery in the last months of my mother's life only because the director of orthopedics had had training that embraced more flexible standards? I suspect that had I not been a physician, I might not have challenged the standards. Similarly, if we had found ourselves in an unknown health system with providers who had been trained differently, choosing this path would have been more difficult, perhaps impossible. They might not have believed I was knowledgeable enough to weigh the options. They might have feared later accusations of malpractice.

I hope that I am wrong, but if I am right about the current state of health care, I hope that our health policies and our health care system will evolve to keep what is good about standards of care in reducing inappropriate variability, while learning to align them with patients' goals and values, particularly at the end of life. This change will require better public education of and increased dialogue about individuals' goals at the end of life.

This shift is beginning, as reflected by the popularity of Atul Gawande's latest book, *Being Mortal: Medicine and What Matters in the End*. Gawande gives a compelling presentation of what it means to strive for "good days" rather than for the often unobtainable potential of more days, no matter their quality. He describes the need for physician training to assist patients and their families in making such decisions. With wider availability of decision support tools for patients and families, more and more physicians and patients are embracing shared decision-making. A decision support tool for patients and families in the management of hip fractures in the elderly would be valuable, especially considering that there are almost 260,000 hospital admissions for hip fractures in people older than age 65 every year in the United States. The one-year mortality for these patients is about 20 percent.

The movement away from fee-for-service payment should better align physicians' choices with the choices of those patients and families who desire fewer invasive procedures, although physicians and the health care systems may also need better assurances against malpractice when shifting standards of care to meet patient circumstances. Our policies and payments must align better with out-of-hospital care, too, including more on-site care in assisted living facilities and flexibility in hospice services. Had my mother been on hospice care when she sustained her hip fracture, for instance, the routine hospice service would not have included physical therapy, although this significantly improved the quality of her final days and likely lowered overall costs. Today, these steps require administrative and medical director assessment and approval. If we begin to make these changes, we can better align the standards of care with the best care, especially at the end of life.

Getting It Right at the End of Life

With the help of a palliative care team, the author's terminally ill mother dies on her own terms.

Dina Keller Moss

At my mother's recent memorial service, lots of people asked to speak. We got to hear from friends and family who had known her from each of the eight decades of her vibrant life. While the details varied, there were important consistencies across all of the wonderful memories that were shared: her great warmth, infinite curiosity, pioneering spirit, and utter inability to tell a joke. But most of all during the formal remarks and informal conversations that followed, everyone in the standing-room-only crowd recalled my mother's fierce independence and drive to do things "her way." And nowhere was this drive better demonstrated than in her determination to go out on her own terms. For this she had needed my help, and I very nearly blew it.

When—just a few days after her eighty-ninth birthday—my mother was diagnosed with a colorectal mass (we would later learn it was cancerous), she restated to me what I long knew to be her fervent wish: no treatment of any kind beyond symptom relief. NO invasive procedures, NO chemo or radiation, NO life-prolonging treatments. NONE! She wanted only one thing: to spend the rest of her days,

Volume 36, Number 7. July 2017.
Editor's Note: The opinions expressed in this article are the author's own and do not reflect the views of the Agency for Healthcare Research and Quality, the Department of Health and Human Services, or the US government.

however many or few there were to be, in her apartment in her lively and supportive community. My job was simply to help make sure her wishes were honored. As it turned out, this was not so simple at all. Just days after the initial diagnosis, despite my mother's long-standing, clearly stated, and just-repeated wish, I found myself reluctantly making an appointment for a preoperative examination with a surgeon for a procedure to reroute her intestine around the mass.

How had we ever come to even consider this?

The Limited Option

For as long as I could remember, my mother had made it clear that she did not value longevity for longevity's sake. Her greatest fear had always been living past the point when she felt good about being alive. "Can you believe it?" a friend or relative would sometimes exclaim in delight about a markedly diminished elderly relation. "She just celebrated her *ninety-sixth birthday*!" In response, my mother would shudder in dismay and reply that she hoped that she would not face a similar fate.

Thus, from the instant she learned about the colorectal mass, my mother told every one of the endless series of doctors who paraded by her bedside that she was really OK with the situation, as long as she could opt to do nothing about it and have a peaceful end when the time came. Though increasingly weak as the days wore on, she remained clearheaded and articulate. And when her voice faltered slightly, or when she got tired of repeating herself, I spoke up for her, and she would nod vigorously in agreement.

Nonetheless, on the fourth day in the hospital, a surgeon arrived at my mother's bedside with a different agenda: to discuss the risks and benefits of two surgical options for addressing the threat posed by the mass. One option was to surgically remove the mass entirely, while a second option involved rerouting the intestine around the mass, which would otherwise be left intact. Since the mass was growing slowly, the surgeon explained, and since there was no sign of cancer anywhere else, my mother was a good candidate for the second, more limited surgery, which was less invasive and promised a speedier recovery.

In fact, the surgeon confidently pronounced my very frail mother an "excellent" candidate for this surgery and predicted a relatively insignificant recovery time with only minimal pain and discomfort. But—oh yes, there was one more thing worth mentioning: the "limited option" involved a colostomy. A hole would be created surgically in my mother's belly, out of which stool would exit into a pouch. The pouch would need to be emptied regularly (once a day or so) to avoid leakage. My mother would need to find a well-fitting pouch to minimize the risks of skin irritation, the extent of odor, and the possibility of leakage. And she'd need to learn to change the bag (it takes practice), adjust her already limited diet, and perform the necessary skin care. Besides this, there would be anxiety about whether the bag would bulge visibly or, worse yet, soil her clothing. Yet the surgeon was certain that with the new technologies and products for colostomies that were available, my mother would adjust in no time.

When I asked what would happen if my mother declined surgery altogether, the surgeon provided a chilling answer. Doing nothing, he told us, would cause her colon to rupture, followed by sepsis. This would be accompanied by acute and possibly prolonged abdominal discomfort and eventually excruciating pain. He painted a graphic picture of what would be happening inside her body to cause this pain. It would be a gruesome way to die. No way would he ever let his mother suffer through that, the surgeon pronounced. His face suggested he was horrified to think that we might even consider it.

In the face of the surgeon's specialized knowledge and the high degree of confidence he projected, our certainty about my mother's long-abiding wish waivered. I, in particular, struggled to reconcile what this expert was telling us with my admittedly vague understanding of the alternative: palliative care.

The surgeon left the room, and my mother began to weep silently. I could not remember when I had last seen her cry, but it had been decades at least. Her hope of a dignified death had been dashed, and she found herself facing a choice between excruciating pain or surgery with a colostomy, with all of the attendant ramifications. She clearly feared she might end up one of the "lucky ones" who "get to live"—in an increasingly physically and cognitively feeble state—to 96!

Probing Questions

I reluctantly scheduled a pre-op appointment for later that month, but I also reached out to a close friend who specializes in research on patient engagement. She encouraged me to probe more deeply the surgeon's predictions and assertions about the likely impacts of undergoing surgery, as well as the consequences of declining it. What exactly did a "relatively easy" recovery mean for an 89-year-old woman who weighed only 118 pounds? How would a colostomy actually affect the quality of her life? Could the pain of a ruptured colon be effectively controlled by a clinician who specialized in palliative care? I sought answers to those questions.

I started by investigating the surgeon's assurances regarding the simple-to-use and odor-free technologies that were available for colostomy patients, since I knew that this would be of particular concern to my mother. We faced the added complication of her Parkinsonism (a condition related to Parkinson's disease that, in my mother's case, left her unable to stand or walk), for which she needed the services of a full-time home attendant.

I called M. R., one of my mother's former aides, who knew her needs, abilities, limitations, and sensitivities at least as well as I did. I trusted M. R. to give me straight answers. I asked if she had had any experience with the colostomy paraphernalia and if she thought my mother would be able to change the bags as easily as the surgeon had suggested. If she couldn't, were home attendants allowed to assist with this activity? God forbid that my mother would have to end up in a nursing home just because of a colostomy.

M. R. assured me that Mom would most likely be able to change the bags herself, though she offered to check on whether an aide would be permitted to help. But then she got to the more central issue: "*You know your mother*," she told me. "You know how much she cares about personal hygiene. She will *not* like the smell. Even if it is not a strong smell, *she* will smell it. They will tell you there is no smell, but I will tell you *your mother* will smell it. It will bother her. *A lot.*"

M. R. went on to describe having cared for an outgoing and sociable retired lawyer who became so self-conscious following his colostomy that he had become a recluse.

For my mother, this would be a truly catastrophic blow. Formerly very active and outgoing, she had already lost a great deal, including her mobility and much of her independence, to Parkinsonism five years earlier. Nonetheless, she remained surrounded by a large cadre of devoted and lively friends—some of whom she had known for decades. When I visited her in the unique Upper West Side community in Manhattan that had been her home for 50 years, we would sit on the bench in front of her building and, without exception, an average of three or four people per hour would stop to sit and chat. Her apartment door was never locked, so friends and neighbors were constantly popping in to play Scrabble, watch a film, discuss a book, or bemoan the deteriorating state of the world.

Over the previous five years, my mother had already begun to feel that her life had been irremediably diminished. Aside from the Parkinsonism, she was growing extremely frustrated with the continuous, if gradual, cognitive decline associated with "normal aging" and the impact it was having on her memory and her ability to use her computer, cell phone, television, and other mainstays of modern life. The prospect of social isolation or other additional losses was more than she should have been expected to bear.

This bleak outlook strengthened my resolve to learn more about whether palliative care could be effective against the specific risks of "doing nothing" as described by the surgeon. The following morning, as my mother was preparing to be discharged from the hospital, a doctor arrived to check her status. We mentioned that she was happy to be headed home and that our next step would be to identify a palliative care specialist who might be able to tell us whether and to what degree the dire consequences of declining surgery could be mitigated.

As luck would have it, the doctor told us that he was trained in palliative care. He immediately validated my mother's decision to reject treatment and offered his unequivocal assurance that she would not need to face an excruciating end. He explained that he could immediately sign her up for home-based hospice, which would include palliative care. This was the first that we had heard of this program.

The Magic Words

Looking back, I can't say whether the surgeon who advised my mother was intentionally engaging in scare tactics. He probably wasn't. Yet his highly subjective, rosy picture of life after surgery and his ghastly view of the alternative were based on his own values, fears, and preferences rather than those expressed by my mother, an elderly woman who above all else feared a longer and increasingly limited existence. Moreover, he was either ignoring, or ignorant of, the potential mitigation of pain and suffering that could be offered through effective palliative care.

Of course, at that moment we were equally ignorant about what palliative care entailed and how effective it could be for those who decline other treatments.

I'll never understand why the option of hospice with palliative care was not presented to us early in my mother's hospital stay, given her very clear statements of her wishes when she was first told of the existence of the mass. It was only when we finally said the seemingly magic words—"we would like to confer with a palliative care doctor"—that we learned that my mother's wishes could in fact be granted. I shudder to think about what might happen to people who are less persistent or do not know what to ask.

I later learned that this omission was not merely an unfortunate oversight but a potential failure to comply with Chapter 331 of the Laws of 2010 in New York State, commonly known as the Palliative

Care Information Act. This law requires that all patients facing an illness or condition that is reasonably expected to cause death within six months be given counseling concerning palliative care and end-of-life options. The New York State Department of Health webpage devoted to the act explains that the purpose of the law is to "ensure that patients are fully informed of the options available to them . . . so that they are empowered to make choices consistent with their goals for care, and wishes and beliefs, and to optimize their quality of life."

The law states that it is the responsibility of the "attending health care practitioner" to provide the necessary information and counseling. In my mother's case, I do not know which of the countless doctors who checked in throughout her hospital stay met that description. Clearly that aspect of the law has to be clarified to produce the desired effect. Perhaps what's needed is the equivalent of a Miranda warning for patients facing terminal illness: you are not required to accept treatment, and if you opt to decline it, a palliative care doctor will be provided for you who will ensure that your pain is fully and effectively managed. But such a requirement would be just the start.

For a law like New York's to be truly effective, hospitals need well-staffed palliative care departments with team members who routinely visit seriously ill patients and who can systematically present palliative care options, both as part of and distinct from hospice. In addition, physicians who treat patients with potentially terminal, or even significantly life-limiting, diagnoses should understand palliative care treatment well enough to be able to discuss it comfortably and meaningfully. Training in medical school and through organizations such as the Center to Advance Palliative Care can help achieve this goal. Otherwise, there will always be situations like the one my mother and I faced, when a patient's choices are inadvertently circumscribed by the limitations of one particular specialist's knowledge, assumptions, or beliefs.

It might not be easy to get practitioners to accept a patient's request for palliative care as a rational and legitimate alternative to more aggressive treatment, however. A colleague who is researching informed consent recently told me that a survey (not yet published) at four hospitals showed that 45 percent of doctors believed that they are in a better position than patients to decide what their patients need.

My mother would have had some choice words for those doctors. She would have pointed to the last six months of her life as evidence of the soundness of her choice. Spared the aftermath of a surgery she did not want, my mother ate and felt better than she had in months. Everyone commented on how well she looked and how upbeat she seemed. She took in several museums and a show. We strolled through Riverside and Central Parks and spent a glorious day at the New York Botanical Garden. She enjoyed visits from friends and family members, including some whom she had not seen in many years. Capping it all was a show of her beautiful watercolors, attended by over a hundred neighbors, friends, and relatives. It was entirely fitting that she chose to donate the proceeds from the sale of her paintings that day to Morningside Retirement and Health Services, a nonprofit organization associated with her co-op whose services had proved invaluable to her as she "aged in place."

Throughout this period, my mother's outstanding hospice team delivered on the promise of compassionate, effective palliative care. The team was careful to include her, her aides, and me in all discussions of her care. They told us what to expect and educated us about what developments might signal the need for a change in regimens. This was certainly not "doing nothing." Palliative care in my mother's case involved active monitoring and managing of her diet, digestion, and medications to maximize her comfort and quality of life. My mother felt engaged, respected, and supported—and she experienced virtually no physical pain.

Slipping Away

About two weeks before her death, my mother began to feel very weak. She became increasingly frail and showed signs of anxiety. She stayed in bed for a couple of days, something entirely new for her.

She called me a couple of times to tell me she was certain that "this was the end." She stopped being interested in visitors and even in phone calls. Then one day she experienced an extremely sharp pain as her home attendant was transferring her from a chair to her bed. The hospice team provided medication that eliminated both her anxiety and the pain.

A few evenings later, I woke her from a nap to ask her if she wanted dinner. She said she thought she might, so I gave her a dose of morphine in anticipation of moving her to the dinner table in another half hour. When I went to get her, she demurred: "Why would I want to move *anywhere* when I am *so* comfortable right here?" Those were her last words. She fell back asleep, and sometime that night she lost consciousness. Over the following two and a half days, in keeping with her wishes, she was heavily medicated as she slowly slipped away.

The evening before she drew her last breath, her nurse stopped in, gently stroked her brow, and spoke to her. Mom showed no signs of hearing her. Her nurse assured us that my mother was in no pain and encouraged me to keep speaking to her, which of course I did. I told her how much I loved her, and that I was truly grateful that she had been so clear about what she wanted. For it was because of the clarity of her wishes, and her steadfast and openly expressed desire to see them honored, that together we were ultimately able to get it right.

The Evolving Moral Landscape of Palliative Care

Deactivating a patient's medical device provides a "good" death, which reflects how perspectives on hastening death have changed.

Myrick C. Shinall

When Mr. S died, it was unusual enough to become the subject of our hospital's monthly ethics conference. After all, it was not often that we deactivated a ventricular assist device (or VAD) in a patient who was awake, alert, and not obviously dying. As I was one of the physicians managing the palliative care unit where Mr. S died, the attendees at the conference were eager to hear my perspective. I could tell that the conference organizers expected members of the medical team involved in his care to describe a sense of moral distress and inner conflict in complying with the patient's request to deactivate the VAD. It turned out, though, that the most interesting part about caring for Mr. S was not the moral distress his decision caused, but the lack of it. As I told the conference, deactivating the VAD was not even the most morally distressing thing I did that day.

Several months before I met Mr. S, his heart failure had entered its final downward spiral. His heart's ineffective pumping and his body's response to it caused more damage to the organ, leading to even less effective pumping and even more damage. It was a vicious cycle that would inevitably lead to his death. He was not eligible for a heart transplant, so he had sought help in the form of a VAD, a mechanical device that served as an auxiliary pump to help keep his blood circulating. It would extend his life and allow him to return home. But without the possibility of a heart transplant, the device would not save him. Eventually even the VAD would not be able to keep his blood moving.

The VAD was meant not only to buy Mr. S more time but also to improve the time he had. The intent was to provide enough pumping power to help him overcome the debilitating effects of heart failure. Unfortunately, the device only prolonged his time in severe heart failure. The VAD and his heart together could get barely enough oxygenated blood to his tissues, so almost any movement was like exercising at maximum capacity. The heart failure also caused his body to retain fluid, which weighed down his limbs and accumulated in his lungs—making it even harder to move and breathe. He spent months suffocating on the fluid his body retained.

Just sitting up was a struggle. Sometimes at home he would lie down on the floor to catch his breath and be unable to get up, even with his wife's help. All she could do was put a blanket on him and hope that by the next morning, he would be rested enough to stand. If not, she would have to call an ambulance to take him to the emergency room. Several times he was admitted to the hospital to receive continuous infusions of medications to make his heart squeeze just a little bit harder, alongside powerful intravenous diuretics to help his body get rid of the extra fluid. The extra life-span the VAD had given him was completely consumed by managing his severe heart failure.

Mr. S knew that the VAD was failing to achieve its purpose, as did his wife, the rest of his family, and the heart failure team that managed him, admission after admission, and kept tabs on him during his increasingly brief outpatient intervals. So it was not a surprise when, during one admission, he decided he'd had enough and asked that the VAD be deactivated. The heart failure team asked our palliative care and ethics teams to consult before acting on this request. It was clear to everyone that he had the capacity to make this request and that discontinuing the VAD was appropriate. He was transferred to our palliative care unit late one afternoon as we prepared to honor his request.

Making Plans

I met Mr. S the next morning on rounds. He was sitting up in bed, looking comfortable and talking with his wife, who sat at his bedside. He looked like an average 65-year-old man you might see on the street, not particularly ill-appearing, until you looked at the IV pole with its continuous infusions of diuretics and vasoactive medications to make his heart pump or the lines leading out from his torso to the controller and battery pack of the VAD. He was talkative and seemed rather cheerful. His wife was harder to read. She looked weary, and there was sadness in her eyes, but no other hint of sorrow in her voice or demeanor.

I introduced myself and began to get to know Mr. S and his wife. They were much more comfortable in the large, airy room brightened by sunlight in the palliative care unit than they had been in the confines of the windowless ICU bay. Without the constant beeping of monitors and bustle of staff, they had both gotten a better night's sleep than they had in a long while. We talked about the family's plans, and I found out that Mr. S's son was traveling to be with him and could not get there until the next day. Our plan was to wait for the son's arrival and then deactivate the VAD. I performed a physical exam, which was unremarkable except for the continuous hum I heard in my stethoscope that came from his VAD and that obscured the faint *lub-dub* of his weakened heart. At that point he looked healthier than any of the other patients in the unit.

Mr. S spent the rest of the day like any other relatively stable patient in the hospital: watching TV, visiting with his wife, and talking with the nurses. When his nurse, his other doctors, and I saw him on rounds the next day, we discussed how the day would unfold. He told us he planned to die that day, speaking as nonchalantly as if he were telling us what he was doing for lunch. His wife had tremendous equanimity about the plan for the day as well. There was a note of relief in her voice. They had moved beyond the point of sadness and were enjoying the remaining time they had together. We counseled them both about the likely course of events after we deactivated the VAD and turned off the intravenous drips: Mr. S would slip into unconsciousness within the next several minutes and die a few minutes after that. We did not expect pain or other bothersome symptoms, but we had medicines ready to administer just in case. We'd give him as much time as he wanted after his son arrived, and he'd let us know when to call the heart failure team to turn the device off. With everyone in agreement, we left him in the care of his bedside nurse and his wife.

Dwindling Moral Distress

After I left Mr. S, I got busy with the rest of the work for the day. There were two patients on ventilators with unsurvivable injuries whom I needed to extubate, and a few other patients who were dying as well. I would need to counsel all of their families about what to expect and monitor the patients for adequate symptom control. I would have to wrestle with the dilemma of whether treating some of the normal but harder-to-watch aspects of dying (the gurgling, fast breathing, and involuntary movements, for instance) was benefiting my patients or simply making their deaths more palatable to their families. I would have to justify to myself that the doses of the medicines I was giving were really for symptom control and not just to hurry the patients' deaths, at the same time as I justified to myself that I had treated the symptoms aggressively enough. As a palliative care doctor, I always feel somehow judged by whether my patients have a good death, which usually means a death that is not too unsettling to the families and nurses. I have to balance this desire to make the death aesthetically pleasing with what I know is my actual duty—to control the patient's symptoms and provide as much comfort and dignity as the disease process allows.

Those balancing acts constitute the moral conflicts that color most of my days in the palliative care unit. Mr. S's case barely registered amid the other care I was giving. I had no worries in his case about symptom control, treating for the family's benefit rather than the patient's, or making the death a good one. Just as predicted, shortly after the VAD was deactivated, Mr. S slipped painlessly and easily into unconsciousness, and his heart stopped beating shortly thereafter. There was no drama, there was no conflict, and there was no suffering. It was odd only in that it was so easy. It was as if Mr. S had an off switch, and we just flipped it.

I was not alone in feeling this way. His bedside nurse told me that it felt weird to have a patient die who was awake and appeared normal while on life support, yet nothing had felt wrong about deactivating the VAD and turning off the drips. The heart failure team said the same thing. It was an unusual case, but not a troubling one.

Our shared lack of distress in discontinuing life support on this patient is truly astounding given what dilemmas discontinuing life support has caused even in my lifetime. Shortly before I was born, the family of Karen Ann Quinlan, a young adult patient in a persistent vegetative state, had to fight the State of New Jersey to have her ventilator discontinued. It was not just New Jersey that objected: many members of the medical profession held terminal extubation (the withdrawal of ventilator support from patients who will not survive without it) to be morally equivalent to murder. A few years later, Kathleen Farrell, who suffered from amyotrophic lateral sclerosis and was competent to make medical decisions, had to seek injunctive relief to be allowed to be disconnected from her ventilator. She died while still on ventilator support as her case was making its way through the courts.

When I was in elementary school, the family of Nancy Cruzan fought the State of Missouri all the way to the US Supreme Court to discontinue the artificial feeding and hydration that they felt Nancy, in a persistent vegetative state following a car accident, would not have wanted. Although the Cruzans failed to convince the Supreme Court to strike down the burden of proof that Missouri demanded they meet in demonstrating that Nancy would have wanted to die, they eventually were able to have the use of her feeding tube discontinued. The attention attracted by the case led to passage of the Patient Self-Determination Act of 1990, which reinforced patients' rights to refuse or discontinue life-prolonging therapy. Now, discontinuing artificial ventilation or nutrition is part of my routine practice as a palliative care physician.

Over time, life-supporting technologies have advanced to include permanent implantable devices such as pacemakers and ventricular assist devices, and health care providers have struggled with the moral dimensions of deactivating those machines as well, which now seem a part of patients' bodies. The culture of medicine, designed to prolong life at all costs, had trouble accounting for the need to stop at some point, and providers acutely felt the clash between honoring a patient's wishes and their own discomfort in stopping life support, which at times felt like murder.

Where to Draw the Line

Looking back, it seems strange that health care providers would ever have been so troubled by things that seem so routine to me now. By the time my medical training took place, famous cases such as Cruzan's had established judicial precedents and generated public awareness, which led to policies that encouraged and empowered patients to make known their wishes about withholding or discontinuing life support and mandated that health care providers abide by them. Advance directives were popularized, physicians began to be reimbursed for having end-of-life discussions, and the specialty of palliative care was developed and formally recognized.

Although these policy changes have hardly made the medical world embrace the concept of limiting or withdrawing medically inappropriate care, they have made such limitation or withdrawal a part of accepted medical practice. The ethical landscape of medicine that I entered was very different than that in which the previous generation of physicians found themselves at the completion of their training. My sense of propriety in end-of-life care is in many ways the product of the policy decisions of the past decades. My comfort in doing things that many compassionate, dedicated physicians found morally repugnant within my lifetime speaks to the power of policy to shape our moral horizons. Policies are not just ways of enacting our moral commitments—they also form those commitments.

The recognition of how much my moral commitments have been shaped by the policy environment in which I trained brings me to the one aspect of caring for Mr. S that troubles me. Compared with the other patients I cared for that day, Mr. S experienced death without the usual clinical or moral ambiguities because he had an off switch that we could just flip. The truth is, every patient I care for has an off switch—the respiratory center in the brain stem—and I know the combination of drugs that will flip that switch.

Despite my best efforts as a palliative care physician, I often fail to make the deaths of my patients as controlled and painless as

Mr. S's. While I wait for their fatal diseases to take their course, I try to alleviate my patients' suffering, but I frequently cannot eliminate it. Many patients and families long for a death similar to Mr. S's, for the quick, controlled resolution to suffering from a disease that will inevitably end their lives anyway. By a quirk of his medical condition, Mr. S had an off switch that our team felt legally and ethically comfortable flipping. Many other patients long for such control over their dying but do not have a device we can deactivate. Witnessing Mr. S's death makes it hard for me to gainsay the advocates of physician aid in dying, who push for policy changes that will make deaths like Mr. S's available for many more people.

Of course, things are never as simple as that. Not every patient with end-stage illness can act as autonomously as Mr. S did, and there are valid concerns that physician-aided dying could be inflicted on people who might not actually want it. Additionally, the course of disease and the chance of recovery might not be as clear-cut in other cases as they were for Mr. S, which complicates decisions about ending a life. Moreover, patients may feel compelled to end their lives because of financial considerations in paying for ongoing care. Nevertheless, we have developed safeguards that help us feel justified in withdrawing or withholding life-prolonging care where we face these same potential concerns about a patient's ability to choose, the uncertainty of recovery, and the extent to which financial concerns are driving treatment decisions.

Yet I feel deeply uncomfortable with the idea of intentionally hastening a patient's death, despite my comfort in withdrawing life-supporting treatment. I cannot help but wonder if my moral disquietude is simply a reflection of a policy environment that insufficiently protects the autonomy of patients with terminal diseases. That policy environment is in the process of changing: six states and the District of Columbia now have legal mechanisms for physician-aided dying, and perhaps more jurisdictions will legalize it in the future. Will the next generation of physicians look back on my squeamishness with a perplexity similar to that with which I look back on those who struggled with the idea of discontinuing mechanical ventilation? At the same time, I believe that there must exist a stable moral framework to guide our actions, regardless of the environment in which we train, and I cannot bring myself to believe that my discomfort with hastening death by introducing rather than removing treatment is purely a result of that environment. So maybe my unease is well founded. Perhaps it is always wrong to kill patients, as the overwhelming majority of the medical field has held until very recently. If that is the case, will policies that enable physician aid in dying blind future physicians to this moral reality? Equally, have the policy changes of the past decades blinded me to the moral realities that the prior generation of physicians saw more clearly? Mr. S's case shows why these policy debates are so intense, for they are debates not only about what we as physicians and patients can do but also about who we are and what we will become.

Necessary Steps

How Health Care Fails Older Patients, and How It Can Be Done Better

A chance meeting between an octogenarian and a geriatrician shows how the US health system focuses on medical care at the expense of older adults' well-being.

Louise Aronson

The clinic was in a dilapidated old building located down the hill from a recently renovated hospital, yet the entryway retained a worn grandeur. Tapering, semicircular walls extended like welcoming arms from either side of the sliding glass doors, and a half moon of sidewalk stretched to the quiet side street.

Volume 34, Number 3. March 2015.
Editor's Note: The woman's name in this essay was changed to protect her privacy.

That's where I first saw her. She stood at the curb with her cane propped on her walker squinting toward the nearby boulevard. It must have been about four thirty in the afternoon then, as I'd asked for the last appointment of the day with the podiatrist doing my pre-op for a minor foot surgery and I was about to be late. The woman was clearly well into her 80s, with a confident demeanor and clothes and hair that revealed an attention to appearance and at least a middle-class existence. She had a cell phone in one hand and seemed to be waiting for a ride.

This was just before Christmas, so when I came back out after five o'clock, night had fallen. But for her tan winter coat and bright scarf, I might have missed her standing in the shadows leaning against the curved wall. She still held the cell phone, but now her shoulders were slumped and her hair disheveled by the increasingly cold evening breeze.

I hesitated. On one side of San Francisco, my elderly mother needed computer help. On the other, our dog needed a walk, dinner had to be cooked, and several hours of patient notes and work emails required my attention.

I asked if she was OK. When she answered yes, I waited. She looked at the ground, lips pursed, and shook her head. "No," she said. "My ride didn't come, and I have this thing on my phone that calls a cab, but it sends them to my apartment. I don't know how to get them here, and I can't reach my friend."

She showed me her phone. The battery was now dead. I called for a taxi with my phone and helped her forward to the curb. She was tired and cold by then and suddenly seemed frail.

We chatted as we waited. Her name was Eva, and she owned a small business downtown—or she had. She was in the process of re-tiring, having been unable to do much work in recent months because of illnesses. She'd been hospitalized twice in the past year, she said. Nothing catastrophic, yet somehow the second stay had dismantled her life. Things had never quite gotten back to normal since then.

The geriatrician in me noted that she had some trouble hearing, even more difficulty seeing, arthritic fingers, and an antalgic gait that favored her right side. But her brain was sharp, and she had a terrific sense of humor.

Finally, the cab arrived. The driver watched as I helped Eva off the curb, an awkward, slow process because of her cold-stiffened joints, the walker, and our bags. As I turned to open the backseat door, he sped away without his passenger. I stared, dumbfounded, and pulled out my phone to call the company and complain. Eva was more sanguine.

"It happens all the time," she said. Just then, a taxi from another company turned the corner. He slowed down for my outstretched hand but saw Eva and screeched off into the night.

"Damn," she muttered.

Doing the Right Thing

It didn't take a rocket scientist—or even a geriatrician—to figure out why taxis didn't want to pick up Eva. Doctors and medical practices often invoke the same reasoning: The old move too slowly, making efficiency impossible. And more often than not, there are complications.

"I'll give you a ride," I said, having refrained from making the offer until then at least in part because of that uniquely American quandary: What if something happens to her and her relatives sue?

Her face lit up. "Oh no," she said. "I couldn't let you do that."

It took almost as long to maneuver her into my front seat as it did to get across town. She directed me to an apartment complex on the steep slope of one of San Francisco's trademark hills. Twin rows of stacked apartments, separated by an expanse of shrubs and trees, rose up the incline like terraced fields, their landings connected by flights of steep, poorly lit steps. As it turned out, Eva lived toward the top. Before we started up, she handed me her keys and pointed, explaining that she needed to exchange her going-out walker and cane for her at-home cane, which was in the garage. Also, she added, it would be a big help if I'd carry her mail.

I phoned my mother to reschedule and called home to say I'd be late. Getting up the steps was slow going. Along the way, I learned that Eva had been to the podiatrist that afternoon because she could no longer cut her own toenails. I told her what I do for a living. We discovered that she got all her medical care except podiatry at my institution and that I knew her primary care doctor and several of her specialists.

As I would write in an email to my general internist colleague the next morning, getting Eva out of my car and up the 49 stairs to her apartment "took nearly an hour because of her grave debility. She is very weak, has audible bone-on-bone arthritis in all major joints, frequent spasms in her left hip, minimal clearance of her right foot and could not move her left foot; I basically had to hoist her." I had no idea how Eva ever made it up the steps unassisted and couldn't imagine how long it might take when she did.

We took frequent breaks so Eva could catch her breath and have a reprieve from the pain she felt with every step. During each rest stop, she told me more about her life. She'd had several romances but no children. Most of her friends were also old and ill, so she didn't see them as much as she'd like. She had lived in the same apartment since the early 1970s, loved it, and would never live anywhere else. She had a blood cancer that hopefully was cured, asthma, some kind of heart problem, and both glaucoma and macular degeneration. After a recent hospitalization for pneumonia, she had been sent to a local nursing home and said she'd rather die than go there again, though she wasn't at all keen on dying. She hated that she could no longer work and couldn't understand why people looked forward to retirement.

Forty some minutes after starting our ascent, we arrived at her apartment. Inside there was a living room crowded with stacks of books, magazines, and mail, and a small cluttered kitchen. It also had what a friend of mine, in reference to her own octogenarian mother, recently referred to as "that old lady smell."

"Shut the door," she said suddenly, but not soon enough. A blur of dark fur grazed my leg, and her cat disappeared down the steps into the night.

We both called him. No response. I walked down the steps, calling and looking. Nothing. After 10 minutes of searching, there was still no sign of the cat. This wasn't the first time he'd escaped, but, she informed me, when an indoor cat got out, you never knew whether he'd be back.

I should have stayed longer to look for him, but I went home.

The Chart Biopsy

Before I left, Eva gave me permission to access her medical record, contact her primary care doctor, and make recommendations to help improve her function and well-being. What I found in her chart speaks with tragic eloquence to some of the fundamental ways in which our health care system undermines both patients and clinicians.

Logging into the electronic record the next morning at work, I learned that Eva had made 30 visits to our medical center in the previous year. This included nine ophthalmology appointments; five radiology studies; four appointments with her lung doctor; four visits to the incontinence clinic; three appointments with her cancer doctor; two emergency department visits; and one appointment each with her cardiologist, a nurse in the oncology clinic, and her primary care doctor. This tally does not include the appointments she missed because, as is noted in at least two places in her chart, "the taxi never showed up." Eva also made frequent phone calls to her doctors' offices and was taking 17 medications prescribed by at least five physicians.

There are words for patients such as Eva and this pattern of care. On the patient side, the words are "complexity," "multimorbidity," and "geriatric." On the system side, they include "fragmented," "uncoordinated," and "expensive." How and why this happens—and it happens far more often than not for all patients, though its impact is far greater on the old, ill, and frail—has at least as much to do with medical training and culture and the economics of medicine in the United States as with the challenges of old age itself.

The notes in Eva's chart revealed clinicians providing thorough, evidence-based evaluation and treatment of the issue or organ system in which they specialized. Sometimes in medicine we see notes that suggest the doctor doesn't really know the patient or is just going through the motions, cutting and pasting from past notes. These notes were different. Eva's doctors and nurses knew her, seemed to care about her, and were applying all of their considerable expertise on her behalf. Unfortunately, their expertise didn't include any of the skills that would have addressed Eva's most pressing needs.

Several notes hinted at what I saw as Eva and I made our slow trek up the steps to her apartment. They documented terrible arthritic pain, significant mobility issues, and ongoing transportation problems. One physician commented that Eva "does not walk much in her own apartment but does utilize a walker. Often, however, she is semi chair bound." Despite these important observations about Eva's most bothersome medical condition and significant life challenges, none of the clinicians seeing her evaluated her joints and gait, did a functional assessment, treated her pain, or referred her to either a social worker or another clinician who might address these crucial needs.

Equally significant were the problems that no one mentioned. No physician commented on the number of doctors Eva had or visits she made, both of which might reasonably raise questions about fragmented care and the need for care coordination. Nor did any of her clinicians address her use of a very long list of medications, a situation known as "polypharmacy" and associated with adverse drug reactions and bad outcomes including falls, hospitalization, and death. Finally, and particularly remarkable for a woman in her 80s with multiple medical problems and no immediate family, no one documented her life priorities and goals of care, or who she would want to make medical decisions on her behalf if she were unable to do so herself.

Over My Dead Body

After exchanging emails with her doctor, I called Eva to tell her what to expect. She wasn't nearly as concerned about her medical care as I was. She liked her doctors and, as is the case for many people, seemed to take for granted that each body part required its own specialist. It also became clear that her medical visits served an important social purpose. When I mentioned that she could get her toenails trimmed by a home-visit podiatrist instead of making bimonthly trips to the clinic where we had met, she exclaimed, "But I've been going there for years. And they're so nice to me!"

I tried to take a casual, conversational tone for my next question and asked whether she'd ever considered moving. I was thinking that a building on flatter terrain, without stairs, and closer to shops would offer her greater independence. Assisted living, if she could afford it, would provide those advantages plus cleaning services, meals, and a built-in social network.

"The only way I'm leaving here," she said, "is feet first."

I didn't press her. As is often the case, Eva's choices made her life more difficult. Yet it was also true that the apartment had been her home for decades, and anywhere she moved would be many times the cost of her 1970s-era rent-controlled apartment. Like the vast majority of older adults, what Eva wanted most was someone who would help her maximize her health and function so she could continue in the life and home she'd created for herself.

Before hanging up, I asked if I could put her on the wait list for our geriatrics practice. I explained that if she agreed, she would get a new doctor who would take a different approach to her care. The geriatrician would manage her diseases as her previous doctors had, but he or she also would begin by establishing Eva's life and health priorities, address her function and transportation challenges, review her medications and appointments to see if all were truly necessary, and be available by phone or to make a home visit if she got sick to try and prevent hospitalizations.

Eva was silent for a moment. Then she said, "That sounds too good to be true!"

What Good Health Care Looks Like

I know most of Eva's doctors. Each one is compassionate, smart, and dedicated. Indeed, her diseases were largely under good control. Yet Eva's health was declining, she was missing appointments, and she was less and less able to care for herself and her apartment. Several of her clinicians recognized this, but none took action. This was not because of personal or professional failings. Most physicians would have taken the same approach to Eva's care as these doctors did. Their actions—and inactions—were the inevitable result of their medical training and our medical system's sometimes myopic focus on medicine at the expense of health.

Medical education prioritizes the same specialties today as it did a century ago, when the average age of death was 47 and when tuberculosis and childbirth were among the leading killers. People in their eighth, ninth, and tenth decades are as different, physiologically and socially, from middle-aged adults as children are, yet all medical students learn pediatrics and adult medicine, but there are no universal requirements for geriatrics training. This makes no sense demographically or medically. There are 48 times more octogenarians now than there were in the first half of the last century, and older patients are the age group most likely to be harmed by medical care. The hospitalization in which Eva's pneumonia was cured, but her life "ruined" by hospital and nursing home time without adequate or appropriate exercise, provides a typical example of how usual adult care fails older patients.

To rectify this situation, two things need to change. First, the groups charged with accreditation of medical schools and residency training programs—the Liaison Committee on Medical Education and the Accreditation Council for Graduate Medical Education, respectively—must mandate training in geriatrics for all medical students and for residents in all specialties where doctors routinely provide care to older adults. Importantly, such training cannot merely consist of providing standard adult care to patients over a certain age. Nor can it be narrowly focused on conditions known as geriatrics syndromes, such as dementia and falls. Instead, trainees must be required to attain competence in the unique approach to care that distinguishes geriatrics as a specialty: individualized, coordinated, team-based care that prioritizes patients' goals, function, and quality of life. Given that the principal source of funding for residency and fellowship training is the Medicare trust funds, it should be relatively straightforward for policy makers to insist on links between graduate medical education payments and training that benefits the Medicare population.

Second, we must have billing codes and appropriate reimbursement for care that improves the health and lives of older adults. Currently, many critical geriatric interventions are either unfunded or funded at such low rates that growing numbers of doctors will not see Medicare patients. For example, a clinician who implemented evidence-based recommendations, such as design of an individualized exercise program or multifactorial intervention, to reduce Eva's recurrent falls—the fifth leading killer of older adults—could not easily or straightforwardly bill for that work. Nor could the clinician bill straightforwardly for assessment and management of Eva's functional status, multimorbidity, goals of care, or caregiver needs and caregiver effectiveness. Moreover, there would be no reimbursement for phone calls with Eva to assess response to treatment changes or troubleshoot her challenges. While Medicare's new Chronic Care Management policy enables billing for time spent communicating with her caregivers, physical therapist, and social worker, the clinician would receive just $41 per month, regardless of how many calls and how much time was required. A system for both services and coordination based on time and with levels of payment that increased with increasing time required would encourage clinicians to provide the care a patient needs instead of providing inadequate care in artificially limited time frames.

A Happy Ending

Eleven months after I met her, Eva finally made it off the geriatrics practice wait list. During her first visit, the geriatrician elicited Eva's health and life priorities and documented the name and contact information of her health care proxy. Because she listed arthritis and pain as her biggest problems, she received steroid injections in her two most painful joints and a pain medication safe in older adults. As her specialists had noted on her recent visits to them, her blood pressure was quite high. It turned out Eva wasn't taking several medications because she hadn't been able to get to the pharmacy for them. She was taking a medication known to worsen incontinence, another shown to benefit middle-age patients but not those older than age 80, and a few that might no longer be necessary. The geriatrician adjusted the timing of her medications so the schedule was simpler and less burdensome and arranged for home delivery from the pharmacy.

Eva's geriatrician also learned that on days when Eva couldn't manage her stairs at all, getting to the medical center was outrageously costly. She had to pay three dollars per step to be carried first down and later back up the steps to her apartment. Since there were 49 steps, this meant $147 each way or $300 per appointment, not including the fare for the ride itself. Fortunately she didn't need to visit the medical center nearly as often as she had been. The geriatrician could treat her incontinence, stable lung disease, and other chronic conditions as well as monitor her for cancer recurrence, all during home visits. Other members of the team—in this case, a nurse, physical therapist, and social worker—helped align Eva's self-management skills, activities, and home environment with her goals. The only specialist Eva still needed was the eye doctor. Equally important, with the money she saved on transportation, Eva could hire more help at home.

Helping an older adult find a caregiver, delineating the caregiver's tasks, monitoring the caregiver's work with the older adult, and ensuring the caregiver's own well-being are not traditional medical tasks. They are, however, among the most important interventions to ensure the well-being and safety of frail older adults. Once in place, Eva's caregiver picked up medications, assisted with cooking and exercise, and cleaned the apartment. She also provided Eva with much-needed social interaction and foot care.

Nearly three years later, Eva is looking forward to her ninetieth birthday. She is frailer than when I first met her, but all her primary goals have been met: she has remained out of the hospital, out of nursing homes, and in her beloved apartment with her cat, who did eventually come home. Those who argue that health care consists primarily of prescriptions and procedures, or treatment of body parts and diseases, have created a system that prioritizes medicine to the detriment of patient health. It's time we took a broader view of health care—one that puts the well-being of patients first and trains and rewards clinicians who work with patients, caregivers, and other health professionals to achieve that goal.

A Family Disease

Witnessing Firsthand the Toll that Dementia Takes on Caregivers

A geriatric psychiatrist recounts the life-changing stress experienced by relatives who care for loved ones with dementia.

Gary Epstein-Lubow

In the summer of 2012, my father-in-law, Ed, telephoned on a Sunday night with some surprising news. Sylvia, his wife of 55 years, suddenly did not recognize him. She had recently been diagnosed with very early-stage dementia, but her symptoms had not yet been this

Volume 33, Number 4. April 2014.
Editor's Note: The names of individuals alive today have been changed to protect their privacy.

severe. Over the phone, my wife and I eventually convinced Sylvia of the truth: Ed was not an imposter. I wished we could stop by their house to help her feel more comfortable, but they lived in New Jersey, and we were miles away in Rhode Island. As a geriatric psychiatrist, I had urged Sylvia to seek care early, which she had done, and so she knew options for her treatment included activities to keep her socially engaged, medication to slow the illness course, and possibly experimental treatment. But on a personal level, I was worried. I worried about Ed, my wife, her siblings, and myself. We would be Sylvia's caregivers for the rest of her life. And I understood the devastating toll dementia could take on an entire family.

Sylvia and Ed

Over the next few months, Sylvia's most difficult symptoms, such as misidentifying her husband, briefly appeared and then disappeared. Eventually Ed discouraged her from driving and cooking so she wouldn't accidentally hurt herself. Generally she accepted her new limitations. She knew she had dementia and agreed to meet with a nurse care manager and a psychiatrist. She was even pleased to have her children visiting more often to help out. But she also had episodes where she'd feel persecuted and frightened. She would get angry. Usually she was happy when I visited, but one day she turned to me, hostile in a way she'd never been, and told me, "You've changed, and I'm very disappointed. It's time for you to leave." I told her I would go after I said good-bye to the rest of the family. A few minutes later, she'd forgotten about it and was happy to have me stay.

This went on for weeks. We tried keeping Sylvia busy with activities she enjoyed, such as outings to meals and the gym. We brought in more clinicians and started her on new medications. But one morning Sylvia was struck with severe terror. Believing Ed to be an intruder, she ran from the house to a neighbor's, who did not understand the situation and called the police. Ed telephoned us in Rhode Island, and we called the nurse care manager, who happened to be planning a visit to their home that morning. The officer and the nurse arrived at the same time. My wife and I took turns talking on the phone with Ed, the officer, and the nurse. The police officer decided Sylvia should be taken to a hospital, so my wife canceled her day's plans, packed her bags, and set off in her car to New Jersey.

The nurse accompanied Sylvia to the ER. It was early in the morning so it was not crowded. Sylvia was given the standard blood, urine, and X-ray tests to determine if any new medical issue might be the cause of her distress. Nothing abnormal was found. Learning I was a psychiatrist, the mental health clinician in the ER called me to tell him more about my mother-in-law.

"Do you think she needs to be in a hospital?" he asked after we had spoken for a while.

"For treatment?" I hesitated. I was not Sylvia's doctor, or really her son. "That's a good question," I said, and explained that my wife would be there soon.

There was a bed available at one recommended hospital, but the doctor wasn't sure yet if Sylvia's behaviors met the criteria for hospitalization. My wife finally arrived, frazzled but glad to be there. As she spoke with her mother, it became clear that Sylvia did not remember the morning's events. She was surprised to hear about it; it even seemed funny to her. When Ed arrived at the ER later, Sylvia was very happy to see him.

Together, our family was forced to face the larger, chronic problems that we'd been wrestling with for months without progress. Hospitalization seemed like the next step. With her family around her, Sylvia understood and accepted the plan. "I have a memory problem," she said. "I'm going to get help."

Hospitalization for Dementia

Sylvia was more confused in the hospital than she had been at home. She started on a ward with psychiatric patients of all ages and then was transferred to a smaller unit of mostly dementia or schizophrenia patients. Sylvia's ending up in the hospital felt to me like a failure—an event that could have been avoided, perhaps, if we had put more services in place earlier, or moved Ed and Sylvia in with us, or selected the right medication, or not selected the wrong medication. I was torn between my belief as a psychiatrist that her symptoms were not so severe and my belief as a son-in-law that our family could not handle any more stress.

At the hospital, Sylvia had no problems recognizing Ed. She relished his visits. They would sit side by side, holding hands, while she confided in him her worries about what was happening around her, telling him she loved him. It seemed as if they were sitting on the porch together again.

A change in her neuropsychiatric medications appeared to be helping. Medication treatment for dementia is complicated, at best. With no drugs approved specifically for the symptoms of dementia, medications for other conditions, such as depression or schizophrenia, are used off-label, with frequent side effects, such as restlessness or sedation. We had tried several before finding something that seemed to help, at least a little.

After a couple of weeks, the family began to worry that hospitalization had only temporarily solved the problem and wondered what we'd do when she was back home. She'd need someone around to guide her, and the job was too much for Ed alone. Our family arranged a call to discuss what would come next for Sylvia, sparing Ed from making the tough decisions alone. We decided for Sylvia's sake to move her to a "memory care" assisted living setting. This left Ed at home alone for the first time in his life. At this point, I wasn't sure which of my wife's parents worried me most.

At the hospital where I care for patients with dementia, I watch these kinds of difficult decisions all the time. But in that moment, being on the inside, seeing how high the stakes were for everyone, it became clear that treatment for the patient with dementia is just one facet of good care. Dementia also takes a toll on the family caregivers—a toll that cannot be discounted.

There are treatments and practices available that could help patients with dementia and their caregivers, including support programs that aim to keep families together at home and to reduce caregivers' burden and depression. Sadly, access to family-based solutions remains limited. In fact, the situation today is not much different than it was when my own grandparents wrestled with the same problems 25 years ago.

Wicky and Irving

My grandparents, Wicky and Irving, were staunchly independent. After Irving retired, they packed the essentials from their New Jersey home and moved 700 miles to be near my mother and her family—my father, me, and my two siblings—in Cincinnati, Ohio, where I grew up. My grandfather, a lawyer trained at Columbia University, was a trusted companion to my grandmother and a loving and supportive guide to my mother, my siblings, and me. In the first years after my grandparents moved to Cincinnati, they spent winters in Florida, competing in bridge tournaments. Irving always took the wheel for the long road trips there and back.

But then Irving started making mistakes. He could no longer keep up in the bridge games, his finances began to confuse him, and he'd forget appointments. Even his movements became slower. As his memory and mobility worsened, he moved with my grandmother to an assisted facility. His gradual decline continued until eventually it became a chore for him to use the bathroom and bathe. When he became incontinent, Wicky, my mother, and Irving decided he would move to a nursing home while Wicky remained at the assisted facility. He did OK at the nursing home. He did not mind clinical staff helping him with washing, bathing, and eating. He enjoyed socializing, and he accepted the simple daily routine.

But Wicky did not adjust quite as well. She visited Irving at least twice a week, and they spoke by phone several times a day. It was stressful and challenging for her, but she knew the value of a devoted marriage. Irving had always supported her choices. She had been an advertising copywriter and also edited a women's newspaper. After marrying my grandfather, she continued to work until she became pregnant with my mother. For decades they had been able to "take care one on the other," a phrase borrowed from Wicky's Russian immigrant mother. But with Irving in a nursing home, Wicky had to figure out how to balance his needs with her own. And as she cared for him and saw his decline, she had to face her own fear of incapacitation.

My grandparents were in their 80s at the time. To Wicky, the man she visited in the nursing home was not the same man she married decades ago. Irving remained, for the most part, accepting and calm amidst dementia's advancing stages. If her own memory ever failed, Wicky told my mother, their only child, she would not be able to tolerate it.

My mother helped Wicky adapt and cope. She planned her parents' finances and living arrangements and became an increasingly central part of their social life, spending more time with them and becoming a closer confidant to her mother. My mother learned to juggle her responsibilities to her parents, herself, my father, and me and my siblings. Then my father was diagnosed with colon cancer, and Wicky knew that my mother had new competing caregiving responsibilities at home.

My grandmother had long worried that she was a burden to her daughter, and my father's cancer only confirmed her fears. She began to think more and more about her own death as a choice. She closely followed the news reports and talk shows that at the time featured Dr. Jack Kevorkian famously helping his elderly patients plan their own deaths. She read his then new book, *Prescription: Medicide, the Goodness of Planned Death*, and discussed it with her family. She often told me how her biggest regret in dying, whenever it happened, is that she would not know "how the story turns out." Then she would add, "But somehow I'll know, and somehow you'll know that I know." That was Wicky, planning to be a loving caregiver, even after her death.

My father's cancer was successfully treated, and Wicky and my mother returned to coping once again with life's challenges.

A couple of years later, Wicky was hospitalized with pneumonia. Her assisted living facility had a skilled nursing unit where she could receive three days of care without any additional charge to her. But she left skilled care after one night, preferring to be in her own apartment. While she was sick, she had been unable to visit Irving in the nursing home, so perhaps getting back to her own apartment would allow her to see Irving again soon.

Wicky was still mostly independent, but being ill must have made her feel afraid that she might soon need more assistance herself. She had always hated the idea of living anywhere other than her own home. She also hated when circumstances dictated what she could and could not do.

Less than two weeks after Wicky was discharged from the hospital for her pneumonia treatment, she committed suicide. The family was shocked. She had acted on what she read from Dr. Kevorkian, ingesting sedatives and alcohol as he advised.

Looking back, I wonder what could have been done to prevent the suicide. Wicky had openly discussed her ideas and feelings about death. On her suicide note, she'd written, "no rhyme or reason" and a comment about her trust that Irving would be OK . . . and then her pen drifted down the page. I am certain her husband's dementia and the toll it took on the family contributed to her decision to end her life. My mother arranged to have Wicky's funeral service in the chapel at Irving's nursing home. My grandfather died a year later.

For the patient, dementia is a terminal illness. For the caregiver, it shouldn't be.

Attention on Caregivers

Caregiving for a person with dementia is a risk factor for homicide and suicide, studies show. Family caregivers of people with dementia have two to three times the rate of depression as noncaregivers—another risk factor for suicide. As time marches on and a patient's condition worsens, the threats for family caregivers continues. My mother had always worried about this. Today my family worries about the same thing: Is caring for Sylvia too much strain on Ed?

A recent Alzheimer's Association report estimated that more than 15 million Americans are currently providing unpaid care to a loved one with dementia. In January 2011, President Barack Obama signed into law the National Alzheimer's Project Act, which led to the publication of the first National Plan to Address Alzheimer's Disease in May 2012. This plan proposes to develop effective treatments for Alzheimer's by 2025, enhance care quality and efficiency, and expand supports for people affected and their caregivers. But the road to reach these goals is understandably long.

A short-term plan is needed, with more attention to families. We need care for the caregivers to be integrated into care for the patients. When Sylvia was in the hospital, I was disappointed (but not surprised) that nobody stopped to ask my wife, or anyone in the family, "How are *you* doing?" When my mother was caring for her father, none of the staff stopped to ask her about herself. After my grandmother's suicide, my mother stepped up her involvement at the nursing home. Each day she would walk out confidently and then sob in her car.

It's tragic that these systems still have not changed. Evidence shows that support programs prevent depression in family caregivers and extend the time a person with dementia is able to live at home. Yet services such as these are still hard to find.

Agencies such as the Alzheimer's Association are helping guide a national agenda while also providing direct local support to patients and caregivers, but we need more federal action to aid families. In the current health care environment, improvements in the integration of patient and caregiver services can be made at initial diagnosis, care transitions, and the end of life.

Policy Solutions

Under the Affordable Care Act, screening for cognitive impairment will be included in annual wellness visits covered by Medicare with no co-pay. As we improve the detection of cognitive impairment, there will be an increased need to assess family caregivers' functioning and to link caregivers and patients to regional centers for family education and resources, which is recommended by most stakeholders.

I wish we'd had a regional center in New Jersey when Sylvia became ill. Instead, we brought her to Rhode Island to meet clinicians I know. We paid out of pocket for a private nurse coordinator service in New Jersey. We were lucky to be able to find and afford these resources; most families can't. Legislation in Congress introduced in April 2011, called the Health Outcomes, Planning, and Education (HOPE) for Alzheimer's Act (S. 709/H.R. 1507), would help make the services we sought, such as care planning, more readily available.

The HOPE for Alzheimer's Act focuses on the time of initial diagnosis. This is an important first step, and similar services for family caregivers are needed when dementia patients are hospitalized or begin residential long-term care. These transitions of care are stressful for family caregivers and are unique opportunities to include them in patient care planning.

A major barrier to these quality improvements in dementia care, including help for caregivers, is a limited workforce. It is expected that in 2030 there will be only one geriatric psychiatrist for every 6,000 older adults with a mental health or substance abuse issue.

An expanded workforce is necessary not only for diagnosis and treatment but also to help family caregivers and patients consider advance care planning, which involves thinking ahead about decisions on medical treatments, housing, finances, and end-of-life care. Access to information about advance care planning is improving, but there is no one place where this process is "owned" over time.

I wonder what Wicky would have thought if one of Irving's doctors or nurses had invited her and my mother to a conference to discuss Irving's end-of-life wishes. I'm sure Wicky would have brought her ideas about assisted suicide—controversial as they were then and today. I imagine how a clinician trained in palliative medicine would have explained to Wicky the hopeful options for a good quality of life, even with advanced dementia. Maybe she would have made different choices about her own life and death. For my family, this is fantasy, but for millions of Americans today, it could be a reality.

Quality of Life

Moving Sylvia to assisted living made Ed worse. After decades of companionship, he now spent most of his time alone. Each day included a burdensome drive to visit Sylvia. He became depressed, and our family turned its attention to him. We helped Ed look at every option for how he could adjust his life to adapt to Sylvia's gradual decline, but nothing, at that time, could soothe the distress he felt with losing Sylvia in his daily life. After a few months, he chose to move to an apartment in the same facility as Sylvia's dementia care unit. We expected this would be temporary, but he liked it and decided to stay so he could be closer to Sylvia.

Now Ed can easily see Sylvia every day, like it's always been. When Ed takes Sylvia "out to dinner" in the main dining hall, or when they visit together in Sylvia's room, he has trouble understanding everything she talks about. "She seems to enjoy it," he says, "and she keeps telling me she loves me."

7

Maternity and Childbirth

Watching the Clock

A Mother's Hope for a Natural Birth in a Cesarean Culture

A physician and mother on giving birth in a culture that increasingly pushes women toward cesarean sections.

Carla Keirns

I had been at the hospital for two days in induced labor, unable to get out of bed or eat, almost 24 hours on an oxytocin drip. Doctors and nurses shuffled in and out of my room, many wearing worried expressions. They wanted to start magnesium for suspected pre-eclampsia, a potentially life-threatening complication of pregnancy, but couldn't prove whether I had the condition because the baby's head was causing bleeding from my bladder. The doctors started to talk about stalled labor, a stuck baby, and going to the operating room. I had assisted at dozens of cesareans when I was a medical student, but I didn't think we were there yet. More time. I just need more time, I thought, as I started flipping through numbers on my mobile phone, looking for friends from medical school who were obstetricians and pediatricians now. I needed another opinion.

As a physician, clinical ethicist, teacher, and health policy researcher, I thought I understood health care in the United States. But nothing in my education or training prepared me for the experience of delivering a baby in the US health care system. As a mother-to-be, I felt what all mothers feel: responsible for the life I was bringing into the world and willing to do anything to increase the chances that I would have a healthy baby. I knew vividly from my time on Philadelphia's busiest maternity ward during medical school that childbirth is an awe-inspiring process when all goes well but can be terrifying if it does not.

Volume 34, Number 1. January 2015.

I became pregnant with my first child at the age of 40. My pregnancy was complicated by diabetes, and dietary changes and exercise proved inadequate to keep my glucose levels optimal for the baby. In my first trimester, I started taking insulin and made an appointment with a maternal-fetal medicine (MFM) specialist, someone who specializes in high-risk obstetrics. When I met the MFM team, I was impressed with their command of the recent literature, their thoughtful rather than reflexive use of technology, and their willingness to admit uncertainty.

Labor is an intricate dance of hormones, muscles, and emotions, usually triggered by the baby when he or she is ready to breathe outside the womb. A few months into my pregnancy, a friend warned me that some obstetricians induce labor in all diabetic mothers early, at 38 weeks' gestation. When I asked one of my doctors about this during an early clinic visit, she assured me that they wouldn't do that.

There was no more mention of induction or the circumstances of my delivery until I came to the clinic for a routine visit at 36 weeks. By then I was coming in once a week to have vital signs and ultrasounds taken. With swollen feet and a round belly, I got up on the exam table. This appointment was with a doctor I had never met before—a middle-aged woman, the fourth member of the MFM group. It was a busy day at the clinic, and she was absentmindedly flipping through my chart as she walked in. She furrowed her brow, looked me up and down, and asked if I had met with the anesthesiologist yet. No, I hadn't been referred. She looked down again and fretted about my sugars and blood pressure, surprised when she saw they were normal. "I hope you go into labor on your own," she said, "because if we induce, the chance of a c-section is 50 percent." I thought of a close physician colleague of mine who, at 42 weeks' gestation, had a cesarean delivery after three days of labor induction. After the visit with the new doctor, I was deeply unsettled, worried that she was already planning my cesarean, the one I didn't want to have unless my baby needed it. A week later I saw the senior obstetrician, who had been managing my pregnancy since the ninth week, and he was much more reassuring.

In the Hospital

On a stifling Monday morning in July, when I was 39 weeks and five days into my pregnancy, my husband drove me to the hospital with a couple of changes of clothes, books to read, and my laptop to watch movies or surf the Web. The doctors were going to induce labor. All of my testing had been normal. But my obstetricians explained to me that the risk of stillbirth increases after 40 weeks, diabetic mothers are at higher-than-average risk, and none of our screening technologies allow us to assess or intervene to prevent it. So almost 40 weeks was their compromise, allowing my baby's body to mature to term but reducing the risk of a catastrophic loss at the end of pregnancy. My sister would be with me at the hospital, updating our parents by phone. They were anxious and excited; this would be their first grandchild.

The induction protocol was a standard strategy of administering two hormones in tandem: prostaglandin to soften or "ripen" the cervix and synthetic oxytocin to trigger or augment uterine contractions. When I arrived at the hospital, I was only one centimeter dilated. The goal for delivery was 10.

Monitors were strapped to my abdomen to assess my baby's heart rate and the strength of uterine contractions. These monitoring devices became available in the 1950s, and by the 1970s and 1980s had become routine in obstetric practice in the United States, often replacing intermittent auscultation, a technique where a clinician listens to fetal heart tones with a fetoscope or a handheld ultrasound. The monitoring helps determine whether the fetus can handle the stress of labor. Research has shown that compared to intermittent auscultation, the use of electronic fetal monitoring allows early intervention when the fetus is in distress, decreasing the rate of seizures from low oxygen and high acid levels in babies, but it does not change infant mortality or cerebral palsy rates. What's more, monitoring increases the rates of cesarean and instrumented deliveries because "nonreassuring" or ambiguous readings lead doctors to intervene to speed delivery. My baby kept moving, and it was difficult to get a consistent reading of the heart rate. The nurses would rush into the room in a panic and say, "We've lost the baby!" My sister found this hilarious, and when they left she would say to me, "I know where the baby is," pointing to my gravid abdomen.

In the first 12 hours after labor was induced, I progressed to three centimeters dilated. I was transferred to labor and delivery for an intravenous oxytocin drip to strengthen the contractions. By morning, my obstetrician measured my cervix at six centimeters using the tips of his index and middle fingers as a guide. He suggested we break the amniotic sac to speed the progress of labor. We both knew that infection rates increase in mothers and babies if delivery does not occur within 24 hours after the amniotic sac is ruptured, but at least I didn't carry Group B strep bacteria, another factor that could have increased the risk of infection in a prolonged labor. When he evaluated me at one o'clock in the afternoon, I was eight centimeters dilated during contractions, and he was optimistic that I would deliver later that day.

When my obstetrician's partner, along with a resident physician, saw me at five o'clock that evening, they found my cervix only four to five centimeters dilated. They suggested that perhaps labor had stalled or regressed. Obstetric textbooks from the nineteenth century discussed regression of cervical dilatation in mothers who are scared or threatened or whose modesty is compromised, but I'd never heard of this in modern obstetrics. I wondered about the accuracy of both of their measurements. It's not as if they used a ruler.

They left me to continue their rounds and returned later with a third doctor, the general obstetrician on call for the night. They said they'd give me a couple more hours. If my cervix was not dilating more quickly, the on-call obstetrician said, "We're going to talk about a cesarean. When things stop, there's usually a reason." They'd said "a couple hours" so casually. I didn't remember until later that active labor is technically not considered "arrested" until there has been no cervical change for two hours during adequately strong contractions, after the cervix is four centimeters dilated.

After they left, I got a visit from a friend, an obstetric anesthesiologist who was on call that night. She asked how I was doing and promised to check on me later. Before she left to see other patients, she looked straight at me and said, "They're looking at the clock. They're not looking at you."

Suddenly I realized I might lose any say in what was happening. Was I at the mercy of doctors who didn't know me and had already made up their minds? I didn't see a compelling medical reason for a cesarean, at least not yet. I thought, "This is what my natural childbirth friends were talking about," when they said women got rushed into surgery they often didn't need.

At that point, I called three friends from medical school—a pediatrician, a family-practice physician who delivers babies, and an MFM specialist. I reviewed the situation with them as I lay in the delivery room, with an intravenous oxytocin drip running into one arm, magnesium into the other, an epidural infusing anesthetic around my spinal nerves, an intrauterine pressure catheter monitoring the strength of my uterine contractions, and a fetal scalp electrode monitoring my baby's heart rate. We all agreed that there didn't seem to be an urgent clinical reason for cesarean. My baby's heart rate tracings were described by the labor and delivery team as "beautiful," and I was tolerating labor fine. My friends counseled patience and advised me to point to the objective data. I resolved to push for more time. My sister watched me open-mouthed. She was shocked by the debate. When I got off the phone with my friends, she said, "I wouldn't know that was a debatable point."

A Subject of Intense Debate

I learned the rest of the story later. At this hospital, the obstetricians, anesthesiologists, neonatologists, and nurses on the labor and delivery team meet twice a day to review the status of each patient in labor. Neonatologists learn when they may be needed at a patient's delivery, anesthesiologists review pain management strategies, and obstetricians and nurses review patients' progress in labor. It was at one of these meetings that I became the subject of intense debate. The MFM physician reviewed the status of my labor and the team's management plan. The intrauterine pressure catheter revealed that although I had been receiving oxytocin for almost 24 hours, my dose had been adequate only for the last two hours. I needed more time. The consensus of the other physicians present—none of whom had actually evaluated me—however, was that I should have a cesarean delivery as soon as possible. The MFM physician later called one of his colleagues at home, lamenting, "Everyone wants to section her!"

Two hours passed, but the physicians did not return to my room. After six hours, I asked my nurse what the plan was, and she offered to get the doctor. I didn't need the doctor, I told her; I just wanted to know what was happening. She said she had been asked to monitor me while they waited to see if I either progressed or developed complications. When she offered again to get the chief resident, I asked her not to.

"If they forget I'm here," I said, "by the time they come back, I'll be ready."

She smiled and left. The labor and delivery unit was busy that night—the doctors were tied up with several cesarean deliveries and an ectopic pregnancy in the emergency department, and I had apparently dropped to a lower priority status.

At six the next morning, the chief resident returned and said, "It's now or never." It had been 21 hours since the amniotic sac was broken. If I wasn't closer to delivery than I had been the night before, it really was time to consider cesarean delivery. She found that my cervix was now more than nine centimeters dilated. I relaxed almost involuntarily when she announced it. It would still be a few hours to full dilation, but labor was certainly not "arrested."

But when the attending obstetrician on call that day visited a few hours later, my heart sank. This was the one I had met at 36 weeks and had hoped not to see again. She announced that I was only four to five centimeters dilated and said we were going to have to talk about a cesarean. I guess she didn't get the report from the chief resident and was still going off the physician's notes from the night before. I said that before we discussed a cesarean, she should confirm the cervical findings for herself. She found that my cervix was more than nine centimeters open. She told me to call when I was ready to have the baby.

I called the team at 11:30 a.m. My cervix was completely open, but I was told not to start pushing until they "got some things ready." I called them back 30 minutes later; I didn't think I could wait much longer. The nurse coached me for the next hour and a half as the baby descended steadily. It was hard going, and I was exhausted. When the nurse saw that my baby's head was visible, she went to get the obstetrician. The obstetrician did not even stop to examine me before she said, "If you haven't delivered by two thirty, we'll have to go to the OR."

"The hell with that," I thought. And in seven minutes, she had the baby in her hands.

But after all that, the medical team wasn't ready. The instrument tray was still in the hallway outside my room. The neonatology team should have been called for my delivery but wasn't. My baby was blue and not breathing. As I lay there, feeling the warm blood flow down my legs, I blocked out all the rest of the sounds in the room, listening for crying. I didn't hear any crying. I barely heard the doctors say it was a boy.

As the neonatal intensive care unit team was summoned to attend to my son, and my placenta was removed manually to slow the hemorrhaging, I was horrified that my physicians had been so unprepared for the delivery. None of the delivery problems should have been unanticipated. Perhaps they really had already earmarked me for cesarean, and the delivery room simply wasn't ready for a vaginal birth.

After we were both stabilized, they handed my son to my husband because I was weak, exhausted, and afraid I would drop him.

What Do the Data Say?

There are circumstances where surgical births are necessary to protect babies, mothers, or both. Obstetrician Ronald Cyr argued in a 2006 paper in the *American Journal of Obstetrics and Gynecology* that an "ideal" cesarean-section rate, such as the 10 percent rate proposed by the World Health Organization, is a myth. It depends upon the specific population's needs and available alternatives. There is, however, broad agreement that the current US rate is too high and not warranted by concerns for fetal or maternal health.

Most commonly used criteria for assessing labor progress in the United States were derived from observations of women in labor in the 1950s. But these observations have come under intense scrutiny recently, in part because of changes in the ages and medical histories of expectant mothers today, as well as changing obstetrical practices. The Consortium on Safe Labor in 2010 published a retrospective study of 62,415 women who delivered a healthy infant vaginally, and it found that the cervical dilatation rate was about half as fast as seen in the 1950s studies. This means that we risk labeling normal labors as slow or abnormal and intervening unnecessarily.

According to a 2011 study in the journal *Obstetrics and Gynecology*, the most common reason for a first or "primary" cesarean in the United States is "failure to progress." A primary cesarean usually means that a woman's subsequent children will be delivered surgically as well. But judgments on what constitutes a slow or stalled labor are often subjective. For instance, a 2012 expert panel of the National Institute of Child Health and Human Development, the American College of Obstetricians and Gynecologists, and the Society for Maternal-Fetal Medicine proposed that physicians should wait 24 hours after administering oxytocin and rupturing the amniotic sac before considering an induced labor "failed," and the clock doesn't start until cervical ripening is completed. The first mention of "failed induction" in my chart was only six hours after the amniotic sac was broken. In March 2014, the American College of Obstetricians and Gynecologists and the Society for Maternal-Fetal Medicine proposed new standards for deciding when labor is too slow or has stopped, suggesting that laboring women should be given more time.

What Happened?

When I talked over what happened later with clinical colleagues, the consensus was, "If you weren't a doctor, you would have been sectioned on Wednesday." Instead, I delivered vaginally on Thursday afternoon. I was lucky to have well-informed physician friends to review the "case" with me in real time.

The principles of "shared decision-making" seemed highly theoretical from the hospital bed. If I hadn't known that more than half of cesareans are for that most elusive of indications, failure to progress, I would have been less hesitant when it was proposed. Besides that, I was naked and uncomfortable, had invasive lines in place, and hadn't slept or eaten in three days. If a doctor I trusted, instead of one I didn't know, had suggested a cesarean 48 hours into my labor induction, I might have agreed. If they had told me that my baby's life or health was in jeopardy, I would have consented to *anything*. The vision of the empowered consumer, or even the autonomous patient, is laughable under these circumstances.

What Should We Do?

Much has been said, written, and done to influence cesarean delivery rates. We should recognize first that if we've been lamenting the increasing rate of cesarean sections since the 1970s, and they only keep rising, then cesareans must be solving some problem. As W. Edwards Deming, an American engineer and business consultant, famously said, "Your system is perfectly designed to give you the results you're getting." Physician Atul Gawande argued in a 2006 *New Yorker* article that cesarean deliveries are versatile in solving a variety of problems that physicians encounter during deliveries, are easier to teach and learn than forceps deliveries, and can be safely mastered by almost any doctor.

Though many groups have called for more use of midwives for low-risk deliveries, this solution doesn't address the growing number of women like me, who are considered "high risk" for complications and, therefore, beyond a midwife's scope of practice.

Some have advocated that obstetricians should be required to get a second opinion from another obstetrician before performing a cesarean, to ensure that the indications for cesarean deliveries are justified. I'm not optimistic that this would help. Few hospitals are likely to have a second obstetrician in-house in the middle of the night, so in practice this would likely devolve into a perfunctory review by telephone. Additionally, physicians who frequently work together may be reluctant to oppose their colleagues' decisions, at least openly.

We've also tried empowering patients with data. The State of New York publishes hospital-level data on a range of obstetrical interventions, based on the premise that data will make for informed consumers. But even if patients are aware of and able to find, review, and understand the data, factors such as geographic access to appropriate alternatives—as in my case—or limited insurance networks of providers may limit patients' use of the data.

In my work as a clinical ethicist and palliative care doctor, I've seen mothers who have lost their babies and fathers who have lost their wives as a result of complications of pregnancy. As a doctor, I don't discount any of the problems my doctors were worried about. I know that our obstetric colleagues are working in territory that is fraught with risk, uncertainty, and liability.

If policy makers hope to change the rate of obstetric interventions—or any other medical tests or treatments—we're going to have to change the culture of medical practice. As expectant mothers become older, with more preexisting medical conditions, guidelines need to evolve beyond those for the low-risk mother in her 20s, and recommendations to avoid cesareans must evolve beyond "choose a midwife instead of an obstetrician."

I already knew, at least in theory, what the risks were when I was wheeled into the delivery room. If we couldn't have an honest discussion about the physicians' fears about my delivery, what hope do we have for shared decision-making with other women? In the end, my son is healthy, I'm fine, and we had the vaginal delivery that epidemiological data suggest was safest for both of us and for any future siblings. Maybe that's enough—it's everything to me and my son—but I think we can do better.

In the "Gray Zone," a Doctor Faces Tough Decisions on Infant Resuscitation

A neonatologist must decide whether to revive a premature baby on the borderline of viability.

Gautham K. Suresh

The newborn resuscitation room was getting uncomfortably hot. The thermostat was set high to prevent a naked, wet, just-born baby's body temperature from dropping rapidly. On this afternoon in May 2004, the neonatology team—the nurse practitioner; nurse; and me, the neonatologist—was finishing up the unavoidable paperwork on a baby we had just resuscitated and stabilized after birth. We were about to leave when a nurse from obstetrics popped her head in, looking flustered. "Don't leave yet," she said. "A twenty-three-weeker just rolled in; she might deliver soon!" With that, she rushed away.

Ron, the neonatal nurse practitioner in the resuscitation room with me, groaned. There was no need for him to say anything. All of us in the room felt exactly the same. A baby born before 37 weeks of pregnancy is considered premature. In general, premature babies have higher rates of complications and death than full-term babies born between 37 and 41 weeks, yet most do well after a few days or weeks

Volume 32, Number 10. October 2013.
Editor's Note: The names of the people described in this article have been changed to protect their identities.

of hospital care. But a baby born at only 23 weeks' gestation has a high risk of dying even with the most advanced life-support techniques. Of the few very premature babies who survive, many end up with severe handicaps, including mental retardation, cerebral palsy, blindness, and deafness. Because of this bleak prognosis, we—the neonatologists, neonatal nurse practitioners, nurses, and other neonatal intensive care unit (NICU) staff who care for extremely premature babies—often face impossible decisions: to provide intensive care to such babies or step back and not intervene.

A Birth and a Debate

The nurse was already on the phone to the NICU asking for additional staff to help us in the resuscitation room. Ron stripped off his latex-free gloves and left to go find out more details about the new mother in labor. I had an ominous feeling. Events were unfolding too rapidly. Under ideal circumstances, the obstetricians would use medications called tocolytics to try to stop preterm uterine contractions. This would give me, the neonatologist, time to talk to the woman in labor and her husband or partner and explain the risks, complications, and treatment choices for a preterm baby. I would try to allay the anxiety and shock that almost all of them felt. With babies born at 23 weeks, because of the high mortality risk—even with intensive care—and potentially poor quality of life, I also would offer the parents the option of "comfort care only." If they chose this option, we would only warm, dry, and wrap the baby and let the parents hold her as long as she was alive. Right after the birth, we would arrange for a baptism or any other religious or cultural ritual the parents desired. The baby usually passed away quickly.

When a pregnant woman arrived at the hospital in advanced labor and about to deliver, however, we didn't have the luxury of time to discuss those options. As I prepared, Ron returned to the resuscitation room, looking tense. Behind him came Mary, an experienced NICU nurse.

"They're not sure of the dates," Ron said. "From the ultrasound, they're saying she could be twenty-three or even twenty-two weeks. She's already six centimeters dilated. Baby's going to pop out soon."

"OK, let's set up, make sure everything is ready," I said, initiating a process that I have learned and honed over nearly 20 years of performing emergency resuscitations. "I'll go talk to the parents; let's see what they say."

I walked into the room next door to meet the expectant mother. The baby would be delivered here and then taken to the resuscitation room where I and our neonatology team waited. There was an atmosphere of controlled urgency in the large, well-lit delivery room— the obstetric doctors and nurses attending to the patient with efficient, practiced movements. She was a black girl no older than 14. Standing next to her was a middle-aged woman, her mother.

This would have been an uncommon scene in my previous job in a NICU in Burlington, Vermont, where the patients were predominantly from a white, middle- or upper-class background. I had recently moved south to Charleston, South Carolina, where most of the patients in our inner-city hospital were black, poor, and socially disadvantaged. I was reminded daily of the huge disparities in pregnancy care and pregnancy outcomes in the United States, where black mothers experience much higher rates of premature birth and black infants die at higher rates than their white counterparts.

The pregnant teenager moaned in pain, an expression of fear in her eyes. It would be nearly hopeless to try to talk to her now. The obstetric resident was performing a vaginal exam to assess how much the labor had progressed and how far the baby had descended. The attending obstetrician—a short, stocky, white-haired man in his 60s named Dr. Carver—hovered near the bed, talking in turn to the patient, the resident, and the two nurses in the room.

I maneuvered past the nurses to the bedside, introduced myself to the girl and her mother, and asked whether they had any questions. The girl's mother shook her head, her face set in a grim expression of pain and confusion. As I walked out of the room to go back to the resuscitation room, Dr. Carver followed me out, closing the door behind him. "She says she didn't know she was pregnant till this morning," he said. The girl had gone to the doctor's office for abdominal pain, discovered she was pregnant and in labor, and was then rushed here to deliver.

I was surprised. Although it was common for women who delivered at our hospital to have received little or no prenatal care, they usually knew they were pregnant. Dr. Carver continued: "The ultrasound from the office this morning says she's twenty-three weeks. We just repeated an ultrasound, and she could actually be more like twenty-two weeks. Anyway, I told the family that you guys will look at the baby when it's born and figure out if it's viable or not."

I dreaded the prospect of having to immediately determine without any reliable medical criteria whether a baby was viable or not. Until a couple of decades ago, physicians commonly used criteria such as whether the newborn's eyelids were fused to decide. At the time, if the baby's eyelids were fused shut and couldn't open on their own, doctors thought the baby wouldn't make it. Research later showed that this test was flawed. Nowadays, the best predictor is a precise estimate of the duration of pregnancy (the gestational age), which is most accurate if the mother reliably knows the date of her last menstrual period, had an ultrasound early in her pregnancy (later ultrasounds are less reliable), or had in vitro fertilization. Unfortunately, many lower-income women don't have access to, or use, prenatal care. For my patient on this day, we had no accurate estimate of the baby's gestation.

Back in the resuscitation room, we began to prepare for the baby's arrival. I sensed disapproval from Ron and Mary, whose expressions, tone, and behavior suggested that they felt we shouldn't be resuscitating 23-weekers whose prospects were so grim. I agreed, but it wasn't up to us. It was for the parents of such babies to decide, armed with the information and advice we provided. So we moved forward. In preparation, the nurse set up a suction catheter to clear the baby's nose and mouth, a face mask attached to an inflating bag to give positive pressure breaths, and a thin plastic tube (an endotracheal tube) to pass into her windpipe to connect her to a ventilator. A medication called surfactant was prepared, which would be instilled through her windpipe into her lungs to help them function better.

By now the respiratory therapist had also arrived on the scene to hook up the breathing equipment. With the whole team assembled, I explained that if the mother wasn't sure of her "dates," 23 weeks was just a guess. We could always withdraw life support after we initiated it, but it would be a catastrophic mistake to let a baby die on a mistaken assumption of her gestational age.

My team did not seem convinced. I knew they felt that they were being forced to do something that they did not agree with. They knew my experience in my previous hospital had been with a quite different patient population. "You know, black patients almost never agree to withdraw life support," Ron told me. Mary agreed—both of them warning that if we resuscitated this baby, we were committed to treating it until the very end, whatever complex form that treatment might take.

From that moment on, things happened fast. The nurse called us back to the delivery room next door. "Baby's coming," she said. We stood next to the mother's bed, waiting for the obstetric resident to deliver the baby. Normally, watching a birth invokes a sense of wonder. To see a new life emerge, to hear the baby's loud cries of protest, to see the vigorous kicking of his limbs and the dawning pink color of his skin as the oxygen floods his body—these moments fill me with a sense of awe, even after witnessing them time after time for nearly 20 years.

An extremely preterm baby is different, however. Most of these babies are born limp and silent as death. Their skin has an unhealthy dark color and is often covered with purple bruises from the delivery. They are so tiny and fragile looking.

The baby emerged quickly, her body slick, covered with amniotic fluid and blood. The obstetric resident lifted the newborn's limp body into the sterile blue towels on Mary's outstretched arms, and we followed her into the resuscitation room, where she placed the baby on the chest-high warm resuscitation bed.

After Ron and Mary dried the baby, I took a closer look at her thin, almost transparent skin, the bruising on her trunk, and her immobile limbs. She looked very premature indeed, possibly even 22 weeks. I quickly estimated her weight as somewhere around 450 grams, about the weight of a 16-ounce cup of soda. Generally, babies weighing less than 500 grams have a really bad prognosis. The outcome wasn't looking favorable for our newborn.

"Start bagging," I said. Ron looked unhappy as he placed the mask over the baby's face and started positive pressure ventilation. Mary reached out to feel the baby's umbilical cord.

"Heart rate less than sixty," she announced after a few seconds.

"The chest's not rising," I observed.

Ron adjusted the position of the mask and tightened the seal of the mask rim, and he was able to get the chest to expand with each positive pressure breath he delivered. The baby was still immobile and blue.

"Heart rate still less than sixty," Mary stated.

"Ron, get ready to intubate," I said. I told the respiratory therapist to take over the bagging.

As Ron prepared to intubate the baby—passing an endotracheal tube into her windpipe to deliver positive pressure breaths—the obstetric resident walked into the room. Clasping her gloved hands together to avoid touching anything unsterile, she craned her neck to look at the baby over our shoulders. "You know, the family does not want any heroic measures for the baby," she told me. "If the baby's going to suffer, they'd rather let her go." It sounded like the obstetric team had more time to talk to the mother about the baby's treatment after she delivered.

"OK, thanks," I replied. "I'll come over to talk to them in a few minutes." I asked Ron to proceed. He slid the thin endotracheal tube into the baby's trachea, and the respiratory therapist gave positive pressure breaths through this tube. The baby's skin, previously a dark shade, was slowly turning pink.

"Heart rate over one hundred," Mary announced.

Dr. Carver checked in on us. "Gosh, she does look like a twenty-three-weeker, doesn't she?" he said, peering at the baby. "Are her eyelids fused?" As if on cue, the baby slowly opened her eyes, drew up her legs, and stretched her arms. The respiratory therapist continued to deliver positive pressure breaths. The baby's skin began to turn a healthy shade of pink, and she was vigorously moving her limbs.

"Wow, she's a fighter," Mary said.

I suggested we perform a Ballard exam, a structured examination of a premature baby after birth in which the baby's muscle tone, skin, ears, and other physical signs of maturity are scored numerically to estimate the gestational age. To our surprise, the exam estimated the baby's gestation to be around 25 or 26 weeks.

The baby weighed 650 grams, much more than any of us had expected. We double-checked and got the same number again. My visual estimate had been wildly inaccurate, and I was glad I had not used it or any other immediate impression to make a snap decision about resuscitation. As the team prepared to move the baby to the NICU for further care, I went to talk to the baby's mother and grandmother. I congratulated them on the birth of the baby girl and explained that she was stable after our resuscitation. We would bring the baby to the mother so she could see her before transferring her to the NICU. The teenager seemed tired, and she did not reply, turning her face away from me. Her mother thanked me but did not smile. Her face was impassive.

The next day I met Dr. Carver in the cafeteria. "How's that kid from yesterday doing?" he asked. She was improving and being weaned off her ventilator support, I reported. He nodded. "I wouldn't have thought she'd make it, at twenty-three weeks, but I guess she turned out to be older," he said.

A Public Health Problem

The baby we resuscitated was one of 15 million premature babies born each year worldwide; that's 1 in every 10 babies born. And one million of these premature babies die each year. A recent report from the March of Dimes ranked the United States (with a 12 percent prematurity rate) 131st among other countries in the world, almost tied with Somalia, Turkey, and Thailand. In the United States, prematurity contributes directly or indirectly to more than one-third of all deaths in infants less than a year old. More than half of these deaths occur in babies born earlier than 32 weeks' gestation, although such babies account for only 2 percent of all births. The estimated cost of prematurity in the United States each year is $26 billion (in 2005 dollars), which includes not just intensive care at the hospital but also ongoing care for long-term problems such as cerebral palsy; mental retardation; visual and hearing impairments; behavioral, social, and emotional issues; learning difficulties; lung problems; and poor health and growth.

So why are so many babies premature? In some cases, babies are intentionally delivered early by doctors to protect the mothers—for instance, if continuing the pregnancy poses a medical risk to a mother with uncontrolled high blood pressure. In our case, the cause was uncertain. No single factor has been pinpointed as the cause of spontaneous premature birth, but many associations have been suggested. Many of these risk factors are social and economic, predating the pregnancy. Rates of prematurity are higher in teenage mothers and twice as high in black women as white women. Maternal smoking, alcohol consumption, low maternal body mass index, age greater than 35, and a short interval between pregnancies are also associated with unplanned premature birth. Women who deliver prematurely are also more likely to be poor and unmarried, with limited education and inadequate prenatal care.

At our Charleston, South Carolina, safety-net hospital, the majority of our deliveries featured more than one risk factor: mothers and their babies with the deck stacked against them socially, demographically, and economically.

"Gray Zone" Babies

Babies born at extremely low gestations are in a special category of their own. Their care raises a host of ethical, moral, medical, and economic questions. Extremely preterm babies strain the limits of neonatal intensive care both technologically and morally.

If you talk to senior NICU nurses and neonatologists, many of them will tell you that 30 or 40 years ago it was common to not resuscitate babies born at 28 or even 30 weeks. Yet over time, neonatal intensive care technology and knowledge improved, and intensive care is now offered at increasingly lower gestational ages.

But with improved ability to save babies, the cutoff point became blurred. Today premature babies around 25 weeks are routinely provided with intensive care because their prognosis is considered good. Babies whose gestation is 22 weeks or less are routinely not offered resuscitation in most hospitals because their outcomes are dismal even with intensive care. Babies in between these thresholds are considered to be in the "gray zone." For them, intensive care is considered to be optional, to be decided upon by the parents after discussions with neonatologists.

Many babies born in the gray zone die within a few days of birth despite maximal intensive care. Survivors usually have long NICU stays with multiple medical problems that often require invasive and painful treatments. After hospital discharge, many have neurologic or pulmonary impairment that affects their long-term quality of life. Caring for such babies engenders much debate and emotional and ethical dilemmas among NICU health professionals, who want neither to provide futile care to nonviable babies nor to sustain significantly premature babies destined for a painful life of extreme disability. In addition, we are aware that NICU care for gray-zone babies who survive but face long hospital stays is costly. Even though we're not supposed to think about "rationing," the burden of the high costs weighs on our minds.

Since the day I started training in neonatology more than 20 years ago, decision-making about extremely premature infants has troubled and fascinated me. Thinking about the baby we resuscitated that particular day, I am reminded of and humbled by how easy it is for doctors to make mistakes when they try to decide which baby lives or dies based on a last-minute ultrasound or how the baby looks in the delivery room. According to a web-based estimator provided by the National Institute of Child Health and Human Development, if the baby girl we cared for had indeed been at 23 weeks' gestation and weighed 450 grams, the probability of her survival without significant disabilities (what we call "intact survival" in our business) would have been around 7 percent. In reality, at 26 weeks' gestation and a birth weight of 650 grams, she had around a 35 percent chance of surviving without significant disabilities. Still a discouraging prognosis, but also a dramatic improvement.

Counseling, Decision-Making, and Challenges

In an ideal world, decisions about the care of these borderline babies should follow the principles of shared decision-making based on in-depth, compassionate discussions between the parents and health professionals before the baby is born. Health professionals should provide information and ensure that the patient understands what is at stake. We must identify the expectant parents' values and preferences; make recommendations if the parents desire; and ultimately help them make choices about when to initiate, continue, or withdraw intensive care.

In the real world, however, expectant parents frequently receive poor prenatal counseling and are not adequately involved in decision-making. Preterm labor usually develops unexpectedly, so patients are frequently admitted emergently under time pressure, when they are sleep deprived, medicated, and anxious. These conditions do not create the optimal setting for conversations about imminent life-and-death decisions.

There is also an issue of health professional bias against extremely premature babies. Multiple studies—including one that I coauthored—have shown that health professionals are overly pessimistic about the outcomes of such infants, overestimating their mortality and underestimating the rates of survival without handicaps.

Neonatologists, obstetricians, and others counseling parents may overtly or implicitly (and often unconsciously) slant their counseling toward nonintervention. Or they may decide whether or not to pursue resuscitation only after they have seen "how the baby looks" in the delivery room. Such practices are not supported by the evidence, but they are common. To help clinicians manage extremely preterm infants, the American Academy of Pediatrics issued a clinical consensus-based report in 2009, which recommends a comprehensive and consistent approach to preterm infants in each hospital, accurate prognostic data for parents, and resuscitation decisions based on the probability of good outcomes with treatment. But there has been no systematic attempt to monitor on a national level how these recommendations are being carried out.

The best solution may lie in preventing premature births and avoiding these tricky ethical situations in the first place. Between 1990 and 2006, despite millions of dollars spent on research to identify preventive measures, the prematurity rate in the United States rose by 20 percent. It reached 12.8 percent in 2006.

Yet recent developments give me hope. The March of Dimes launched a campaign in 2003 to prevent prematurity by raising awareness of the problem, disseminating evidence-based practices and assigning prematurity rate "report cards" to states. The campaign also aimed to improve women's access to medical care during and between pregnancies and sponsored research on prematurity prevention. In 2008, the March of Dimes extended the campaign until 2020 while also expanding the effort globally, with activities in 62 countries by 2012.

By 2011, the prematurity rate in the United States had declined to 11.7 percent.

In addition, the Centers for Medicare and Medicaid Services launched a national initiative in 2012 called Strong Start, testing whether enhanced prenatal care for women enrolled in Medicaid or the Children's Health Insurance Program can reduce premature births. Healthy Start, a program from the Health Resources and Services Administration, funds efforts to reduce the infant mortality rates and improve perinatal outcomes in the areas of highest need. The program has shown promising improvements.

It is my hope that these kinds of programs will ultimately reduce premature births and the number of gray-zone babies who are born. As a result, neonatologists will face fewer snap decisions such as the one I had to make in the delivery room that day, and babies, their families, and society will benefit.

Reversing the Rise in Maternal Mortality

A mother's death in the 1950s tears a family apart; 60 years later, maternal mortality is on the rise again.

Katy B. Kozhimannil

In the fall of 1997, I drove an hour from my college to the small rural town in central Minnesota where my grandmothers lived to pay them what I thought would be a routine visit. The first stop was at my Grandma Lorraine's. She'd left necessities out on a table for me: a $20 bill, a martini, and a note inviting me to join her at the casino. I decided instead to walk the six blocks to my Grandma Rita's house.

Grandma Rita lived in a one-story two-bedroom yellow ranch house on a corner, less than a mile from where she was born. Next to the home's garage was a vegetable garden with half of a bathtub

Volume 37, Number 11. November 2018.

painted blue inside and set up as a grotto for a two-foot statute of the Virgin Mary.

It was my first time sleeping over at my grandparents' house as an adult, without my siblings, parents, or cousins. My grandpa had gone to the basement to do a puzzle, and I recall the warmth of the kitchen light as my grandma and I sat around her small, round kitchen table that night. The table was covered with a plastic gingham tablecloth, and on it sat the usual: two stacked plastic containers of cookies, the top one filled with homemade ginger cookies and the bottom with store-bought sandwich cookies. The walls were decorated with "fancy" plates that my grandparents had mounted—gifts from friends or relatives who had gone to far-off places like Niagara Falls. In that cozy, familiar kitchen I heard a haunting story. I knew that my grandma's sister had died young and unexpectedly, but that evening as darkness fell, I heard the whole story of how maternal morbidity and mortality had shaped our family.

On December 28, 1947, Grandma had traveled 30 miles from her home in the countryside to give birth at a regional hospital in the largest city in Stearns County: St. Cloud, Minnesota. Her baby was stuck, and she spent four days in hard labor. Then she endured nearly a day of pushing, pain, and bleeding before she lost consciousness. My Uncle Tom was finally born on New Year's Day, 1948, and both of them were hospitalized for two weeks after the birth.

"I don't remember anything from that time in the hospital," Grandma whispered, eyes downcast. Still, she said, she was grateful that the hospital had the capacity to care for her and her baby. It could have been worse.

After Tom came, my Aunt Becky, and then her third pregnancy, which ended in a miscarriage. Her third child, my mother, was born in 1952.

Beattie

Three years later, in 1955, Grandma's younger sister Beatrice, whom she called "Beattie," headed from a stint as an army nurse to a job in a Choctaw tribal jurisdictional area in Oklahoma. She got pregnant shortly thereafter with her fifth child, a daughter who would be named Jeannie. When she went into labor, she traveled off the reservation to give birth because there was no local hospital with maternity services. Beattie never left the hospital after giving birth to Jeannie. She died within days, from what was likely a pulmonary embolism—a blood clot in her lungs.

Beattie was 29 when she died, leaving her five children behind. Her husband was unable to care for them but wanted the children to stay together. Grandma Rita, with three small children of her own, could not adopt all five, but she wanted to adopt the girls. Her other sister, Millie, offered to adopt the boys. That way, at least the children would be raised in the family. Still, Beattie's husband insisted the children should stay together, and someone outside our family eventually adopted them in a closed process.

"Back in those days I thought about Beattie's babies every day . . . every day," Grandma told me. "When I fed my kids, I wondered who was feeding my nieces and nephews. I wondered if they were hungry. I also wondered if they knew about their mother."

In the early 1970s, our family finally reunited with Beattie's five children, after the oldest child successfully searched for us. They had been raised by a family in northern Minnesota, not 200 miles from their aunts, uncles, and cousins. Putting the pieces of our family back together was emotional for everyone, punctuated by joy at what we had regained and sadness about what had been lost forever. It feels like a small miracle that I now see one or two of Beattie's children at family reunions, but the pain of the earlier separation never fully abated.

That night back in 1997, I lay awake in Grandma's guest bedroom. The last photo taken of Beattie sat on the nightstand: a professional photograph of my great-aunt in her army nurse uniform and matching white hat, her dark hair carefully arranged in curls, her gaze slightly to the right of the camera. Looking at her gentle smile, I replayed the horror again and again. I was grateful that Grandma Rita had trusted me to hear this. I would not discuss Beattie's death and her children's separation from the family with Grandma Rita again in depth until days before her death, but the family silence had been broken.

Beattie was one of about 1,800 women who died giving birth in the United States in 1955, when the maternal mortality rate was approximately 47.0 deaths per 100,000 live births, according to historical vital statistics records. During the 1960s and 1970s, access to health care and the quality of health services improved, and maternal mortality decreased. In addition, family planning improved dramatically as birth control became widely available and abortion became legal. Medicaid was established in 1965, and in an effort to improve birth outcomes, a separate eligibility category for pregnant women was added in 1984. Clinical innovations such as the development of safe surgical birth by cesarean further improved health outcomes for mothers in the United States. More hospitals were built, and perinatal care was regionalized. These factors all contributed to massive improvements in maternal health. By 1978, the year my mom gave birth to me, the maternal mortality rate had dropped to 9.6 deaths per 100,000 live births. Maternal mortality in the United States reached its lowest point in history in 1987, when 6.6 women died per 100,000 live births, according to the Centers for Disease Control and Prevention. That year about 250 US mothers died giving birth.

When Grandma opened up to me about our family's trauma, she had reason to hope that the darkest days for new mothers were in the past. Birth was safer for her daughters than it had been for her. So why, by the time I was giving birth to my own children, did that change? Since the conversation with my grandma in which I truly understood, for the first time, how maternal mortality had shattered the lives of those I loved, I focused my professional work on maternal health.

Maternal Mortality on the Rise

In the 1990s, the maternal mortality rate in the United States began to increase. Between 1987 and 2010 it more than doubled, reaching 16.0 deaths per 100,000 live births. But as the rate ticked upward, the trend was not making headlines. In graduate school in the 2000s, I learned that childbirth was the most common and costly reason for hospitalization, yet it was not routinely studied. Shockingly little was known about safety and the quality of care in childbirth, and shockingly little attention was paid to the women who died, or nearly died, giving birth.

Blame for the recent rise in maternal mortality falls upon the policies and systems that do not support the health of women before they become pregnant, during pregnancy, at the time of childbirth, and postpartum.

Notably, some of the trends that accompanied the prior decline in maternal mortality have begun to reverse course. From the late 1980s through 2009, the percentage of reproductive-age women who reported being uninsured at some point during the prior year increased substantially. Even for those with health insurance, maternity care became more costly, especially with the rise of high-deductible health plans, and many women experienced gaps in health insurance coverage during the postpartum period. Access to reproductive health services has declined—a trend that is associated with more restrictive laws and policies enacted in the 1990s and 2000s. Hospitals and clinics have closed or consolidated services, and shortages in the maternity clinician workforce have affected access to care, practice arrangements, and relationships between patients and their care teams. Additionally, fee-for-service payment models have incentivized procedures over physiological processes in childbirth, and some of the medical procedures that were developed to support safe childbirth—such as labor induction and cesarean delivery—became overused when not medically necessary.

By 2010, when I gave birth to my daughter, the US maternal mortality rate was worse than that in 56 other countries. I would have been statistically safer giving birth in Egypt, Iraq, Latvia, Mongolia, or Uruguay than here. That year, the US maternal mortality rate was the highest it had been in decades. Nearly 1,000 women died giving birth, and more than 60 percent of these deaths were likely preventable, according to a 2018 analysis by nine state maternal mortality committees. In the United States, no group bears this burden more heavily than black mothers, who are more than three times as likely as white women to die giving birth and—if they survive—more than twice as likely as white women to bury their babies before their first birthday. In addition, rural mothers are more likely than urban mothers to lose their babies to infant mortality. They have to travel farther to receive care during pregnancy and childbirth, putting both them and their babies at risk. The perspectives of the people, families, and communities who have endured the greatest losses should guide policy responses to maternal mortality in the United States.

Reversing the Rise

A mother's death is a searing, unimaginable tragedy, the effects of which last for decades. In this country we cannot turn our backs on our mothers. The United States must take action to prevent needless deaths among women who have just given birth. To do so, I believe, will require drastic improvements in five areas: data on maternal deaths and near misses, access to care, birth equity, accountability, and—most importantly—listening to the mothers who were nearly lost and the families left behind by maternal death.

The first step toward making childbirth safer again is the establishment of a national maternal mortality review committee and support structure for consistent data collection within and across states so that we can understand how each maternal death fits into broader patterns of risk. Other countries do this and are able to respond quickly to emerging crises in maternal health. Only about half of all US states have maternal mortality review committees. I've served on

Minnesota's committee since 2012. Every six months we meet to discuss maternal deaths in the state, reviewing every bit of evidence available (from clinical records and autopsy reports to obituaries) to determine whether the death was preventable and to try to draw broader lessons from patterns that emerge across stories. To my knowledge, the data from our work in Minnesota have never been publicly released, and our numbers are too small for meaningful statistical estimates. It's heartbreaking to know that our work has little influence on the rising tide of maternal mortality. This should change.

Second, access to care must improve. Health insurance coverage before, during, and after pregnancy helps women afford the care they need. Recent efforts to repeal portions of the Affordable Care Act that require health plans to cover maternity care as an essential benefit threaten financial access to care during pregnancy, and Medicaid eligibility policies that drop pregnancy-related coverage 60 days after childbirth contribute to health insurance "churning" in the postpartum period. Also, women need access to care in their own communities whenever possible. To keep maternity units open, policy efforts to address workforce shortages and the financial challenges of low-volume obstetrics are needed. More than half of rural counties currently have no hospital that provides maternity care, and in those communities there is a need for housing and transportation support for mothers who travel to give birth in distant communities—as well as for emergency response support locally.

Third, we must directly confront the unconscionable racial disparities in maternal death. To do so requires a recognition of the role of racism—at an interpersonal level and at a structural level—in creating or denying opportunities for health, including the chance to flourish during pregnancy, childbirth, and early parenting. Key to this work are efforts aimed at improving workforce diversity and addressing unconscious bias among clinicians and within health care institutions. A recently published Council on Patient Safety care bundle provides concrete guidance on steps that clinicians and health systems can take to reduce racial disparities in care during pregnancy and childbirth. But the work of improving racial equity in childbirth extends well beyond the health care system to encompass the social determinants of health, including employment, housing, education, food access, environmental health, and criminal justice—all of which require policy-level action.

Fourth, in childbirth, it is essential to hold health plans, health care delivery systems, and clinicians accountable for what matters and to make it easy to do the right thing. The development and use of evidence-based tool kits and protocols can improve the safety of clinical care for every birth. California provides an instructive example through the efforts led by the California Maternal Quality Care Collaborative, which has successfully deployed care protocols that have led to demonstrable reductions in maternal morbidity and mortality. Additionally, payment reform that prioritizes outcomes over procedure use holds potential for reducing the financial incentive to overuse services.

Finally, and most importantly, reversing the rise in maternal mortality requires listening to mothers. It is not sufficient for mothers to be present: they need to be front and center in the decision-making in each of the areas described above. Women's questions and concerns about their health and safety during pregnancy, labor, delivery, and postpartum must be heard. The onus is on health care delivery systems and those individuals who are clinically responsible for care during childbirth and afterward to find ways to heed every warning.

Reversing the rise in maternal mortality is possible, and California has the track record to prove it. From 2006 to 2013, California bucked the national trend, and maternal mortality declined by 57 percent, from 16.9 deaths to 7.3 deaths per 100,000 live births. Many of the ideas outlined above come from California's experience, and that state gives me great hope. At the same time, potential policy decisions on the horizon could pose a threat to maternal health. Efforts to roll back the Affordable Care Act threaten to dramatically reshape and scale back state Medicaid programs, which finance nearly half of all births nationally. Furthermore, court decisions and policies restricting access to family planning and abortion services threaten women's health and disproportionately affect women who are medically underserved, including those in rural, low-income, or black communities.

"It's a Shame What Is Happening to Our Moms"

In 2017, Grandma Rita was 94 years old and living in a nursing home, where she was receiving hospice care. Twenty years had passed since she'd told me about Beattie. On her bedside table, she kept an article cut from a newspaper: a *Washington Post* op-ed I'd written with a colleague about the challenges rural women face to give birth.

I was proud of the article, which had been picked up on social media by members of Congress, but I was prouder still of the attention it garnered at the nursing home in rural central Minnesota where my grandmother lived. She showed it to every nurse, doctor, personal care attendant, food service staff member, clergy, family member, and volunteer who walked through the door of her room.

On a cold day in mid-December 2017, I drove across the windswept prairies to visit Grandma, bringing my own daughter with me. It would be the last time I spoke with her. On her windowsill, not one foot away from the tattered copy of the op-ed I'd written, was the last picture taken of Beattie, in her nurse's uniform. It was the same photo that I remembered from that evening two decades ago in Grandma's old home. Grandma looked at the picture and said, "You know . . . my sister Beattie . . . I miss her every day. I think about her every day." She touched the well-worn piece of newspaper lightly and said, "It is important that moms get the care they need. I am so surprised about how many places have no hospitals. It's a shame what is happening to our moms. I could have died if I had not been able to get to a hospital when I gave birth."

Grandma Rita died four days after my visit.

I have Grandma Rita's nose, her love of books, and her pathological sense of responsibility. On June 20, 2010, exactly 61 years after she gave birth to her second child, I gave birth to mine, also a daughter. I named her Rita.

The stories I tell my daughter Rita about her great-grandmother reveal the fragility of life and the depth of women's strength. If we can turn the pain of maternal death into righteous indignation about the loss of something so precious, we can take action to ensure that for our daughters and granddaughters every birth is sacred and safe.

8

Opioids and Substance Abuse

- Down the Rabbit Hole: A Chronic Pain Sufferer Navigates the Maze of Opioid Use   *Janice Lynch Schuster*

- In Opioid Withdrawal, with No Help in Sight   *Travis N. Rieder*

- The Fine Line between Doctoring and Dealing   *Pooja Lagisetty*

- Intoxicated, Homeless, and in Need of a Place to Land *Otis Warren*

Down The Rabbit Hole

A Chronic Pain Sufferer Navigates the Maze of Opioid Use

A woman living with chronic pain tries to manage her condition while maneuvering through the maze of opioid medications.

Janice Lynch Schuster

I have never been one to visit my primary care physician regularly. For many years I kept healthy, with periodic visits to local urgent care facilities for my minor health care woes. By 50, though, I had accumulated my share of problems and had found my way to specialists who could help me along: an orthopedist for my arthritic knees; an ear, nose, and throat doctor for my poor hearing; and a dermatologist for occasional instances of squamous cell cancer. Even so, I considered myself to be among the mostly well.

But in the winter of 2013, I began to experience a terrible and persistent pain in my tongue. It alternately throbbed and burned, and it often hurt to eat or speak. The flesh looked red and irritated, and no amount of Orajel or Sensodyne relieved it. I paid a rare visit to my doctor, who suggested I see my dentist, who, in turn, referred me to an oral surgeon. He thought the problem was a result of my being "tongue-tied," a typically harmless condition in which the little piece of tissue under the tongue, called the frenulum, is too short, limiting the tongue's range of motion. It seems I have always had this but had never noticed because it hadn't affected my ability to eat or speak. Now things had changed. The doctor recommended I undergo a frenectomy, a procedure to remove the frenulum and relieve tension on the tongue.

"Just a snip," he promised.

It sounded trivial, and I was eager to be done with it. Although I make a living writing about health care, I didn't even bother to Google the procedure. It never occurred to me that "a snip" might entail some risks. I trusted the oral surgeon. His medical and dental degrees gave me confidence in his skills and knowledge.

And so in March 2013, a day before I was due to travel to Chicago for a week-long business conference, I went in for the frenectomy. I sat back in the dental chair and, as I have always done, closed my eyes lest I catch sight of what I imagined must be an exceedingly long novocaine needle.

My calming thoughts ended abruptly with the first novocaine shot, dead center in the floor of my mouth. I nearly fainted with pain. By the second shot, I was in tears, grasping the surgical aide's hand in distress.

The procedure began and although my mouth was numb, the slicing sounds of the cut made me anxious. It felt as if the oral surgeon was, in fact, slicing my entire tongue away. When I thought the ordeal was surely over, it proved to be only halfway there, as he still had to sew up the wound—a task that required several stitches to the underside of the tongue itself. The oral surgeon and I were both surprised at how painful the process had been for me. Even when he was done, I continued to cry.

He prescribed routine follow-up care: salt water rinses and an antibiotic. And Percocet, a fairly common painkiller, for when the numbness wore off.

Down the Rabbit Hole

I had optimistically expected to be back to normal in time for my flight to Chicago the next morning. But that evening, when the novocaine wore off, the intense pain returned. I took the Percocet. When that didn't help, I added aspirin and then dutifully swished with warm salt water, all to no avail. I called the oral surgeon to explain that my mouth was killing me. He prescribed Norco, a slightly stronger medication than Percocet, and I picked it up from the pharmacy. Norco was a bad match. It left me itching from head to toe. On my way to the airport the next day, I stopped at the CVS to get yet another prescription painkiller, but this one made me vomit. I boarded my flight anyway, certain that I'd feel better at any moment.

But over the next few days, the pain worsened. It was a combination of sensations, alternating between the feeling that I had scalded my tongue, bitten down on it hard, or pierced it with something sharp. No matter what I did, it hurt. In the ensuing days, my oral surgeon called in a variety of medications, none of which helped. I managed to get through my talk at the conference by sucking on ice chips.

Later the following week, still in terrible pain, I went back to the oral surgeon, whose colleague suspected that an undissolved stitch was triggering my pain, and removed it. That didn't help either.

The Root of the Problem: Nerve Damage

Though I did not know it then, my misery had just begun. In the ensuing months, I would become one of the estimated 100 million American adults who live with chronic pain. In my case, the pain was eventually characterized as neuropathy: pain caused by nerve damage. Although the course of neuropathic pain varies by source and mechanism, and treatments range from sophisticated surgical interventions to massage, the outcome is often the same: the chronic pain itself becomes an affliction to be treated, in addition to whatever injury or condition caused it in the first place.

Invisible pain is hard for others to understand. If I'd broken my leg, for instance, I could have propped up my foot or limped around on crutches. Neuropathic pain is far less evident. As far as oral pain goes, there is little to be done. And little, really, can be done, to let others know you suffer from mouth pain. Yet such pain is constant: you cannot simply put your tongue up or not use it for a while.

Severe chronic pain can make life itself a test of endurance and will. People who suffer from chronic pain—and who turn to physicians to heal it—often discover that some clinicians view us with skepticism or disbelief. At times we are reduced to begging for help. Even then, many of us are dismissed as drug-seeking addicts.

For several weeks after my return from Chicago, I was in nearly daily contact with the oral surgeon, who said again and again that he had not heard of a patient experiencing such pain as a consequence of a lingual frenectomy. And yet when I began to Google relevant terms—tongue damage, tongue pain, frenectomy, and so on—I found repeated references to the kinds of damage that can occur. Eventually, I joined a closed group on Facebook, where I met a few hundred other people who were suffering from mouth pain, triggered for the most part by routine oral surgeries.

I had now entered the maze of pain management, where getting effective medication that I could tolerate, and an adequate supply, itself became a constant struggle.

At one point, when my oral surgeon was away for a week, his assistant refused to call in a refill of pain medication. This was in 2013, before newer regulations were enacted that would have prohibited such a prescription from being called in. According to the surgeon's electronic records, I already had been prescribed a veritable pharmacy of pain meds and had received more than 100 pills over the course of the month. The electronic record did not include my bad reactions to several of these nor that I could not take them as prescribed.

The surgeon's assistant finally agreed to order a refill once I had returned any unused medications to the office or to the pharmacy. Unfortunately, it turned out that the office could not accept my unused pills, nor could CVS, which had no collection mechanism in place. The pharmacist did, finally, call the doctor to verify that I had at least tried to return the pills. Finally, the new prescription was filled.

More than a month after my surgery, the pain had become even worse. Some days I could hardly get out of bed; I was so incapacitated by pain and its companion, despair. The oral surgeon called on his colleagues and, eventually, I wound up at the University of Maryland School of Dentistry, seen by an oral surgeon who specializes in oral and maxillofacial surgery.

He injected two points in my jaw with novocaine. The relentless pain subsided almost immediately—an indication that, in fact, the pain was originating somewhere in the tongue itself, and not in my brain.

The surgeon told me he suspected that an errant stitch had wrapped around a nerve in my tongue. Although exploratory surgery was possible, he said, it was unwise, as the nerves were so small and the process so likely to cause more damage. Left on their own, he continued, the nerves might heal in 12 or 18 months. He suggested I find a neurologist to explore appropriate treatments.

Eventually I found one who could actually see me, but I was dismayed when she handed me a few samples of antidepressants and antiseizure drugs, both indicated for the treatment of neuropathic pain but both likely to cause troublesome side effects. It was up to me to select which I'd prefer—a choice that worried me, since neither seemed a good solution. I saw another neurologist, who suggested a trial of Cymbalta, an antidepressant that might lift my mood and relieve my pain. It could take six weeks to kick in.

And so, week after week, I continued to see my own oral surgeon, who would dutifully examine my tongue and lament my ongoing need for painkillers. I had told him about my lifelong problems with depression and my ongoing treatment for it, and he was concerned that I might be predisposed to addiction. I assured him that the opioids had no salutary effect on me—I certainly didn't feel euphoric, as some apparently do—other than to take the edge off the pain long enough for me to get through each day.

Risks and Benefits of Opioids

Like most US clinicians, my oral surgeon and other health care providers have reason to be concerned about the safety of long-term use of opioid analgesics, such as Percocet and Oxycontin. First touted as a godsend for the management of severe and chronic pain when the Food and Drug Administration (FDA) approved it in 1995, Oxycontin has since become a widely abused medication. Contrary to claims by leading advocates for better pain management, Oxycontin can, in fact, lead to addiction. It undoubtedly leads to physical dependence, and those who take it routinely cannot simply quit.

In the mid-1990s, Russell Portenoy emerged as a champion of opioids for use in managing moderate-to-severe pain for a range of medical conditions. Until then, they had been used almost exclusively for advanced cancer. Portenoy pointed to research that, he claimed, indicated that patients would not abuse opioids but would limit their use to managing pain. Today's opioid epidemic tells a different story.

Since the introduction of these drugs, there is no denying that millions of suffering Americans now have more effective options for pain management. But the cost of this improvement has been the emergence of a widespread public health crisis of addiction and fatal overdoses. Figures from the Centers for Disease Control and Prevention (CDC) indicate that in 2010 some 12 million Americans were using prescription painkillers without a prescription. The CDC reported that in 2008 painkillers played a role in as many as 15,000 overdose deaths—more than heroin and cocaine combined. In addition, as regulations have been tightened to control Oxycontin and other prescription painkillers, more and more people have resorted to heroin and other illicit drugs.

In the fall of 2013, the FDA took back-to-back actions that reflect our confused national response to opioids. On October 24, 2013, the director of the FDA's Center for Drug Evaluation and Research announced that the agency would recommend tightening regulations that govern how hydrocodone is prescribed, making it harder for people to acquire it. The very next day the FDA approved a new extended-release opioid, Zohydro ER—despite recommendations by its own technical advisory committee that the drug presented such significant risk of abuse that it should not be approved.

In the realm of chronic pain, such competing and conflicting aims are the norm. Pain patients like me often feel trapped between the clinical need to treat and manage pain and the social imperative to restrict access to such drugs and promote public safety.

Widespread access to opioids for every single ache and pain is clearly not the answer. In a 2011 report, the Institute of Medicine (IOM) calls pain management a "national challenge" that will require "cultural transformation" in terms of researching pain to understand its scope, particularly in terms of its underdiagnosis and undertreatment. Among the IOM's recommendations are that providers and patients alike receive more education on the ways in which biology and psychosocial factors affect the experience of pain. For me, understanding and accepting those factors has not done much to alleviate the day-to-day experience of pain.

The IOM also recommends that providers "tailor care to each person's experience" and promote self-management of pain, which could include strategies such as keeping a pain journal; monitoring pain triggers; and learning coping strategies, such as meditation and yoga. Experts also recommend that primary care doctors coordinate care and treatment with pain specialists. When my primary care doctor dismissed my symptoms, I wound up trying to organize and coordinate my care as I journeyed among my oral surgeon, neurologists, pain experts, primary care doctors, and psychiatrists. It was more complicated than I could manage. During a two-week period last summer, I wound up in the emergency department four or five times because of adverse reactions to several medications.

One of these visits occurred early in the course of my ordeal, after I had a severe reaction to Cymbalta. I had not been warned that it could make me photosensitive, and as a fair-skinned person, I was at even greater risk for this. When I erupted in giant welts, I called my dermatologist, perplexed by what was happening. As I sat in her examining room, I fainted, and she called 911.

It was terrifying to leave the dermatologist's office on a gurney. I remember the cool rain that fell and how the EMTs shielded my face from it. I remember their urgency and their calm as they got an IV going and tried to get my vital signs back to normal.

At the emergency department, the doctor stood near my head, patting my arm as he looked at my chart, then saying, "I see that you are in chronic pain."

"I am," I said, crying.

"And are you depressed?" he asked. "Because I have never met a pain patient who was not."

To be sure, the complex interplay of mind and body affects how one experiences pain, as well as how it is treated. No doubt, clinical depression simply makes one feel worse and makes it even more difficult to try alternative and complementary pain treatments. In my case, I had little energy for anything.

Waiting for Better Days

I have since explored alternative therapies: herbal remedies, guided meditation, journaling, and exercise. These lift my spirits but do not reduce the near-constant presence of pain.

There is still a chance that my pain will vanish—for instance, if the nerves do heal in the next few months. If they don't, then I have a lifetime ahead of me to adjust to this situation.

I do my best not to let pain run my life. Some days are better than others. I try to keep a sense of humor. Some days, though, are hard to endure, and I chide myself to be grateful that I am still standing.

Had I spent a moment or two researching the risks of the frenectomy, would I have avoided this experience? Perhaps. But now I have few choices but to live through it.

I am weary of this experience. When I am not overwhelmed by pain, or depressed by it, I am furious at the attitudes I encounter, especially among physicians and pharmacists. It has been stigmatizing and humiliating. The cost to my productivity has been steep, and the toll on my family has been high. I have spent countless hours in doctors' offices, and even more hours in bed. Some people find meaning in suffering, but I find none.

I read science news closely, hoping that some new nonnarcotic pain treatment will yield better and more effective treatments that do not include the risk of abuse and addiction. In the meantime, though, pain sufferers like me swim against two tides: the pain itself and the experience of seeking treatment for the pain. Pain represents a complex nexus of mind and matter. Surely, for all our yearning to understand both, we can find better ways to ease the suffering and devise treatments and strategies that do more good than harm and that do not shame and stigmatize those who suffer.

In Opioid Withdrawal, with No Help in Sight

A patient receives prescription opioids after an accident—and no support from his physicians as he weans himself off.

Travis N. Rieder

On May 23, 2015, my motorcycle was struck by a careless driver in a large van. My left foot was crushed, the great toe and first metatarsal shattered, while pieces of the first, second, and third metatarsals exploded out through the top and bottom of my foot. My first hospital stay lasted eight days. There, the orthopedic trauma surgeon saved my foot from the immediate threat of amputation and sent me home with a vacuum-assisted closure device for the wound, while the plastic surgeons figured out how to close the large hole on the bottom of my foot. After a week, I was admitted to a second hospital for a skin graft, but the surgery was aborted because of the size of the wound, and I was again sent home with a vacuum-assisted wound closure device. Finally, I was admitted to the limb salvage center at yet another hospital, where a team of surgeons performed a "free flap," transplanting skin, fat, muscle, vein, and nerve from my thigh to my foot. The surgery lasted nearly nine hours and required five

Volume 36, Number 1. January 2017.

days in the intensive care unit plus another five days on the general care floor.

By the time I went home, I had been in and out of hospitals for more than four weeks.

I had been heavily medicated since the day of the accident—with varying degrees of success at relieving the pain—with both immediate-release and extended-release oxycodone, as well as intravenous morphine, fentanyl, and Dilaudid (hydromorphone). Having been opiate-naive prior to the accident, I found this to be a confusing, dreamy, and sometimes scary time. Even when I was home between surgeries, I wasn't really present for my family—either for my one-year-old daughter or for my wife, who was somehow holding our family and home together in the aftermath of the accident.

After the transplant surgery, my previous drug regimen was not keeping my pain under control, and the hospital's pain management team was brought in to consult. The attending physician upped the dosage of oxycodone, added intravenous acetaminophen for two days, and prescribed gabapentin, a neuropathic pain medication. My pain was finally under control, so long as I continued to up the doses as I became tolerant—which my various doctors were always happy to do.

Tolerance and Physical Dependence

I know that some of what happened next was my fault: I'm well educated, and I should have been thinking more long term. But if I'm perfectly honest, I was just scared. The memory of those early days in the hospital was constantly present, and my life revolved around keeping my pain manageable; whenever I began to feel like I was losing control, I upped the dosage and informed my doctors, who wrote a new prescription. It never even occurred to me that I should be aggressively looking for the first possible moment that I could begin decreasing my medication, and no one told me to do so.

It was nearly August before my original orthopedic surgeon, at an X-ray follow-up, asked about my pain and noted that I ought to think about getting off the meds. He seemed surprised that I was still taking such high doses, and his recommendation to back off had an air of admonishment about it. He did not, however, have any suggestions, nor did he mention that I might have difficulty quitting. He simply told me to call the plastic surgeon to get advice on weaning. The plastic surgeon advised what I now know to be a very aggressive taper, which involved dropping one-quarter of my daily dose of extended-release oxycodone and gabapentin each week for the following month and using the immediate-release oxycodone only when I absolutely needed it. My wife—a research scientist—was skeptical of the approach, but we assumed that my physician knew best. That night, I reduced my first dose.

A Glimpse of Withdrawal

The first week of tapering I became nauseated, lost my appetite, and began to have difficulty sleeping. I spent most of my days lying on the couch, waiting for time to pass. When the symptoms began to improve around day six, however, I assumed that my body was becoming accustomed to this process.

But then it was time to drop the next dose. During that second week, I ate even less and began spontaneously crying. The crying was disconcerting by itself, but after a few days it would launch me into depressive episodes. Each day felt a little worse, and I began to believe that I would never recover. My body, my brain, my hormones—they all felt so profoundly *broken*. We called my doctor, who focused on the intestinal problems, advising stool softeners and lots of fluids. When I meekly pushed him about my overall discomfort, he told me that if it was that bad I could just go back on the meds for a while. But I felt too invested in the plan, nearly two weeks into this misery, and I committed to sticking it out.

At the beginning of the third week, things started to go off the rails. The discomfort that had been keeping me awake at night turned into what I would come to call the "withdrawal feeling." It felt like being on fire inside, with muscles that restlessly twitched. I stopped trying to sleep in my bed. Instead, I never left the couch, napping for 90 minutes at a time. I alternated between sweating and being covered with goose bumps, and I had several crying spells a day. The depression was crushing. My wife called the doctor again. He told her it might be time to go back on the meds now. When she asked if there was anything the doctor could prescribe to ease my symptoms, he said that he wouldn't advise me on the matter any longer, as he was clearly out of his depth. Officially, he recommended that I go back on the meds and find someone else who was more comfortable dealing with opioid dependence. But the thought that the nearly three weeks of suffering I'd endured might have been for nothing, and that I might have to go through it again in the foreseeable future, was unbearable. I decided to stick to the plan.

After I took my final dose of opioids at the start of week four, I thought withdrawal might kill me. The nausea left me curled up on the floor of the bathroom in the middle of the night because I couldn't get to the toilet quickly enough on my walker. I went three days without real sleep and—for the very first time in my life—had suicidal thoughts.

My wife began calling every doctor who had treated me, and none would help. Several said only that I should go back on the meds (with no advice for after that); others told me to find pain specialists; and one told me to go to the emergency department, where they would probably put me back on medication until I stabilized. The pain management team that had treated me in the hospital refused to see me, saying that they were an inpatient team and could prescribe narcotics but did not treat withdrawal. We called every doctor in the area with similar results. I found an independent pain management clinic, and they said the same thing that the hospital team had: they could prescribe medication but couldn't treat my withdrawal symptoms. They advised my wife to take me to a methadone clinic.

We finally found a clinic that said they would help to manage my withdrawal, but the next available appointment was five days away.

"It's an emergency," I told the woman on the phone.

She told me I should go to the emergency department then; all she could do was put me down for the end of the week. I thought to myself (and I think I believed it) that I would be dead by then, and I hung up.

Day three without sleep. I had not left the couch. By this time, my wife was scared. She asked me to refill the lowest-dose prescription I had. It had been nearly four weeks of absolute misery, and I had been without any prescription pain medication for six days. I desperately wanted to make it out the other side, but I had started to doubt that there was one. I refilled the prescription. That night, I went to bed instead of staying on the couch and put the meds on my nightstand. I told myself that if I was still awake in four hours, I would take a dose. An hour later I was asleep, and I didn't wake up until morning.

I had come out the other side.

A Failure of the Medical Community

No one will be surprised to hear that I was angry. Angry at myself, angry at my doctors, angry at the medical community. Just— *angry*. I had been hit by a van and undergone five surgeries, yet the worst part of the experience was my month in withdrawal hell. How could it be that my doctor's best tapering advice led to that experience? And how could it be that not one of my more than 10 doctors could help?

I have since learned about some strategies that help patients get free from narcotics. For instance, I now know about appropriate weaning schedules, such as tapering off each medication separately, at a rate as low as a 10 percent drop per week. I've learned about Suboxone (buprenorphine and naloxone) as an alternative to methadone for weaning patients off narcotics, as well as a variety of medications for managing the symptoms of withdrawal, such as trazodone for insomnia and clonidine for restlessness. So why aren't these strategies common knowledge among physicians? *Shouldn't* they be?

It seems clear to me that they should. Physicians are the gatekeepers of medication for a reason: they are supposed to protect their patients from the harm that could come from unregulated use of those medications. Physicians, public health officials, and even the Centers for Disease Control and Prevention tell us that we are in the midst of an "opioid epidemic" due to the incredible addictive power of these drugs. Yet when people become addicted to painkillers after suffering a trauma, the best advice they might get from physicians when coping with withdrawal is to go back on it to feel better. Can we really do no better than that?

A Moral Principle for Prescribers

I understand that I might have gotten unlucky and that many physicians could have done better by me as a patient. But no one should get as unlucky as I did. I believe each physician has a duty to prescribe only those medications that he or she can responsibly manage for the length of a patient's need, including the treatment of foreseeable side effects. If a physician prescribes a highly addictive medication for pain management, with serious and predictable withdrawal effects, then he or she has a duty to see that patient through the weaning process as safely and comfortably as possible. Or, alternatively: he or she has a duty to refer the patient to someone who will be able to see the patient through that process.

I am an ethicist, and it seems to me that such a principle is well supported by bioethical reasoning. Indeed, this can be seen simply as a specification of the principle of nonmaleficence or the Hippocratic oath to "first, do no harm." By prescribing a drug that has predictable harmful effects without a plan for dealing with them, a physician is at least partially responsible for causing those harms.

Now, one could object that physicians cause harm all the time in this way, as many medications and treatments have harmful side effects that are accepted as the cost of care. Chemotherapy, for instance, certainly harms the patient, but we do not condemn oncologists for prescribing it.

The objection doesn't stick, however, because we *should* condemn oncologists if there are methods for managing the side effects of chemotherapy that they do not prescribe alongside the treatment. Indeed, as our ability to treat certain chemotherapy-related toxicities has advanced, we have come to expect that cancer patients receive this care. In short, we already accept this ethical principle. If a physician opens up a patient to predictable harm—even for very good reason, such as saving the patient's life—the physician must do what he or she can to minimize that harm.

Structural Implications

The medical system is organized in a way that makes it quite difficult for physicians to live up to their withdrawal care responsibility, as my experience illustrates.

The most obvious problem is educational. To responsibly prescribe opioids, physicians must have the relevant information concerning dosing, dependence, weaning schedules, and symptom management. There is mounting evidence, however, that medical schools are not making this a priority. Judy Foreman, in her powerful book *A Nation in Pain*, surveys the literature on medical education only to find that there is little to no formal training in pain and pain medicine in US medical schools. For context, she notes that Canadian-trained veterinarians receive, on average, far more education on pain than do US medical students.

Of course, pain specialists do receive such training. Yet the two pain management teams from whom I sought help delineated their jobs as prescribing pain medication, not helping patients withdraw. Methadone clinics, meanwhile, deal largely with maintenance and detox programs for people with long-term addiction, not necessarily someone in my situation. In my case, the nonspecialists, the pain specialists, and the addiction specialists all failed to see routine withdrawal care as falling within their purview. Given the physiology of dependence, we know that a number of patients who are prescribed opioids will require this kind of care. As a community, we need to decide whose responsibility these patients become.

In team-based medicine, particularly when acute care has chronic implications, it is often unclear who "owns" the patient at any given time. Although I had a prescribing doctor, the fact that he was one of a dozen physicians who were seeing me might have diluted his sense of responsibility. This likely affected every aspect of my care, from education (whose job was it to teach me about the dangers of opioids?) to a general lack of coherent planning for dosing, monitoring, and ultimately withdrawing. *Somebody* must take responsibility for long-term pain management for patients like me, or many of us will simply fall through the cracks of the complex medical system and either suffer the harms of unsupervised withdrawal or wind up addicted.

Learning from This

The plastic surgeon who had been managing my prescriptions eventually apologized and admitted that he simply had not known how to deal with opioid dependence. I hope that he committed to learning more after this experience.

My goal is not, however, to change one doctor's view about what he owes his patients. Instead, I want to start a broader conversation about physician responsibility for opioid-related harms, as well as the systemic forces that make it easier or harder for physicians to recognize and discharge their responsibilities. Opioid withdrawal isn't minor. It's not "just temporary" or "the price to be paid" for pain relief. It's not morally innocuous. The moments that I was in withdrawal— all of the *thousands of moments* of genuine suffering—were the worst of my life. That kind of suffering *matters*, and its seriousness needs to be reflected in the way we deal with prescription opioids.

The Fine Line between Doctoring and Dealing

To treat a patient with addiction, a physician must overcome feelings of frustration and betrayal.

Pooja Lagisetty

Gary first came to see me a few years ago, walking in with a swagger in his step and greeting the entire staff with high fives. I was starting my internal medicine residency training at a community health center in Boston that served a large number of patients with opioid-related addictions, and Gary was one of my first patients. He was in his 50s and thin. His shirt was tucked into jeans that were too large, loosely fastened with a belt that was too big. His clothes were stained but not soiled, and his tattoos, both professional and homemade, camouflaged his track marks.

He looked surprised when he met me. Perhaps it was my youth or that I didn't fit his stereotype for a physician. He didn't look like my typical patient either.

Gary was well prepared for our appointment, reciting the details of his medical history with ease. Although he had failed interferon therapy for his hepatitis C, the disease was under control, and he was waiting to take one of the newer medications that had fewer side effects. He pulled out crumpled papers from his pockets: records from another hospital with results from an extensive work-up of his heart.

Gary had long struggled with addiction. He had used more than $100 worth of heroin mixed with crack cocaine and benzodiazepines every day for the past 30-plus years. I didn't want to overstep the boundaries of privacy on our first visit and ask him where he got the money for it. All I knew was that he lived in public housing and didn't currently have a job. When I asked about his family, he quickly responded, "They cut me off."

Volume 36, Number 1. January 2017.
Editor's Note: The patient's name has been changed to protect his privacy.

He had been treated at multiple detox programs and rehabilitation centers without success, but he remained willing to try anything to quit using. He was meticulous about using clean needles and had managed to escape the scary diseases, such as endocarditis and HIV. In addition, he carried intranasal naloxone, a rescue medication that could be used to reverse an opioid overdose in an emergency. Despite his carefulness, I was afraid for his health. There had been three fatal overdoses in our neighborhood in the past month. There were rumors that the heroin that had recently started to be sold in the area was laced with fentanyl—a synthetic opioid analgesic more potent than morphine—which can make heroin even deadlier.

Gary spent most of our visits talking about how he would do anything to quit using and how carefully he managed his chronic medical issues of hypertension, reflux, and hepatitis. I referred him to a mental health addiction specialist located within our clinic, and we discussed getting him on the wait list for a methadone program, the recommended treatment option for someone with Gary's long history with opioids and high tolerance for the drugs. Methadone treatment centers, which administer methadone to lessen the symptoms of opiate withdrawal and block the euphoric effects of opiate drugs, were sparse and in high demand. Gary would have to wait months to get in. In the interim, he showed up to every primary care visit to get refills on his blood pressure meds, and only once did he come to the clinic intoxicated.

"Doc, I need help," he said that day, barging into the room, drunk and high. He could barely make it through a sentence, his voice slurred from the alcohol and heroin, but his body pacing quickly back and forth. At least he had had the mental clarity to come to the clinic for help.

I got him to the emergency department and placed in a detox unit. He called me eight days later, and with a booming voice said he was doing better. Unfortunately, he was still on the wait list for a methadone program. As with so many other patients in this situation, I was about to lose this opportunity of sobriety to intervene.

This was when I first considered starting Gary on buprenorphine.

The Promise of Buprenorphine

Buprenorphine was one of the few medications a primary care physician like me could prescribe in a primary care setting instead of in a specialized clinic. It is an opioid partial agonist, which means that it produces euphoric effects that are weaker than those of heroin and methadone. The drug's opioid effects also level off at a moderate dose, which lowers the risk of misuse and dependency. The Drug Addiction Treatment Act of 2000 permits any licensed physician who completes an eight-hour course to obtain a waiver to prescribe buprenorphine in office-based settings. This law opened up the possibility for physicians without specialty training in addiction or psychiatry to treat patients for opioid use disorders.

Because buprenorphine can be administered in a primary care physician's office, patients can avoid much of the stigma attached to being treated in specialized addiction facilities. Patients can pick up monthly prescriptions at local pharmacies, self-administer the medication, come in for monthly appointments, and manage their disease in much the same way they would manage any other chronic illness.

Gary was not the ideal patient for buprenorphine though. He was still using multiple other substances, including alcohol, cocaine, and benzodiazepines. Buprenorphine mixed with alcohol or benzodiazepines could precipitate a life-threatening interaction or a fatal overdose. A structured methadone program with daily counseling and check-ins was likely more suitable for him. But I also knew that every day that I waited to start Gary on treatment, as I debated whether he was the perfect patient for buprenorphine or if buprenorphine was the perfect drug, was another opportunity for Gary to overdose out on the street.

So after Gary completed his latest stay in a detox program, I offered him buprenorphine at our next office visit.

"Doc, I am willing to try anything, if you think it will work," he said.

Because I was still a resident and had not yet completed the eight-hour buprenorphine course to obtain a waiver, my attending physician wrote the prescription, and we initiated treatment. For three weeks I remained hopeful as Gary passed his urine toxicology screens, showing no evidence of illicit drug use, and attended his mental health counseling appointments, which were encouraged for patients undergoing buprenorphine treatment. The urine screens and check-ins with me provided feedback and reinforcement to help Gary stay on track. Before initiating buprenorphine, Gary would intermittently see the mental health specialist, but tying the prescription to counseling incentivized him to attend the appointments more regularly.

Not a Miracle Drug

Gary did well on buprenorphine for almost an entire month and seemed optimistic about the potential for recovery. But at his one-month visit there was no evidence of buprenorphine in his urine toxicology screen—only heroin and oxycodone. I performed a search of our state's prescription drug monitoring program database to see if any other providers had given him oxycodone and found not one but two other doctors doing so. My heart sank. I felt so duped. He had never complained of physical pain to me or asked me to prescribe him oxycodone. I wondered if this was all part of a carefully constructed plan to have multiple providers prescribe him different medications with street value. I confronted Gary and saw the muscles in his body tighten.

"Doc, the prescriptions were for a friend," he said. He denied using any of the drugs for himself.

"Maybe somebody slipped me some oxycodone," he added. "Please believe me."

I told him it was too risky to continue the buprenorphine since he was still using other substances. I considered the possibility that he was selling the buprenorphine to buy other street drugs. Suddenly, the room felt so small. Gary jumped up quickly and paced from corner to corner, texting on his flip phone. I debated standing to stop him from pacing or hiding myself away behind the computer that separated us.

"So this is it," he stammered.

A part of me wanted to reach forward and touch him, and another part of me wanted to fold my arms and give him the sort of firm, disapproving glare that I had last seen from my parents as a child.

I stood and nervously placed my hand on his shoulder. He gathered his belongings and stormed out with no response.

Physician or Enabler?

When Gary was using *street* drugs, his addiction was a problem that I could so easily compartmentalize. Heroin was a bad habit that happened behind closed doors or on the street, outside my clinic. However, when he was using *prescription* drugs, I, as his physician, became accountable. I suddenly felt like I was his enabler—and his dealer.

I can't think of any other medication that puts physicians in as precarious a situation as opioids. While we try to reduce harm, many of us fear we are indirectly fueling an epidemic. I didn't learn about this feeling in medical school. Addiction was killing my patient, and I could not shake the feeling that he had betrayed and deceived me.

Ultimately, I had to realize that this was not about me but about Gary. I reminded myself that all of my visits with Gary prior to finding out about his positive urine screen for opioids had helped him. Every visit offered him a safe space to talk about his social and physical problems. My patients with other diseases, such as diabetes, also often didn't take their medication as I prescribed. "Medication nonadherence" was a term that frequented primary care charts and rarely evoked any feelings of betrayal and rage. If anything, we were taught to dig deeper into why our patients were nonadherent (medication costs or limited health literacy, for instance) and find shared solutions. Why did I take Gary's nonadherence with buprenorphine so personally? I needed to have the same resiliency in treating Gary that I was hoping he would have in overcoming his addiction.

As a resident physician, still in training, I was fortunate to have the support of incredible mentors who helped answer my questions and self-doubts around Gary's care. I decided to give him a call, but there was no answer. After some time, I wrote Gary a letter letting him know that I would always support him and that my door was open.

Six months after I wrote the letter, he returned to see me, greeting me with a high five.

"Doc, I was angry with you." He gave me a toothy grin. "But I got your letter."

Getting Help

People like Gary need help, but access to addiction treatments such as methadone maintenance is poor. Buprenorphine provides a primary care–based option for physicians to tackle the disease. While buprenorphine treatment failed in Gary's case, it's had great success in others. In a 2015 study by Jennifer Potter and colleagues in the *Journal of Substance Abuse Treatment*, almost 50 percent of patients on buprenorphine were no longer using opioids at 18 months. Today, only about 33,000 physicians (less than 3 percent of all physicians) hold licenses to prescribe buprenorphine. By contrast, almost all physicians are licensed to prescribe opioids for pain. Doctors often cite logistical barriers as the main reason for not taking on the work prescribing buprenorphine. Many clinics lack the infrastructure to support the frequent appointments, urine toxicology screens, and mental health counseling recommended for buprenorphine treatment. I could have cited similar logistical concerns as a reason to stop treating Gary and patients like him. However, I must also admit that I was scared. I didn't know how to help Gary without adding fuel to a public health epidemic. Furthermore, his failures could have deterred me from continuing to treat patients with opioid use disorders following my residency if it weren't for the support I received from trusted mentors.

Given the promise of buprenorphine for many patients, we should encourage more physicians to obtain waivers to prescribe it. In

July 2016, President Barack Obama signed into law the Comprehensive Addiction and Recovery Act, which proposes $62 million per year in new funding for the next five years to combat substance abuse and reduce overdose deaths. Also in July, the Department of Health and Human Services finalized a rule change that increased the number of patients that physicians with buprenorphine waivers can treat, from the current maximum of 100 patients to 275.

But given physicians' reluctance to obtain buprenorphine waivers, it is unlikely that these policies will fully achieve their goals without concurrent efforts in medical schools to provide educational support to address the psychosocial tension that comes with treating patients with addiction.

Physicians who treat patients with addiction need support. Many medical trainees and physicians have limited access to experienced providers who can teach them about how to successfully prescribe pain medications, provide support as patients are tapered off of opioids, and help treat and support the patients who become addicted. My own interest in addiction as a primary care physician stemmed from my role models during medical school and residency who showed me just how powerful harm reduction can be. I was fortunate to be trained in a clinic where four of my attending teachers were skilled in prescribing buprenorphine. Not only did they provide me with emotional support when Gary relapsed, they also reminded me just how difficult and daunting the burden of addiction continued to be for Gary. Of course, changing how we teach the finer art of doctoring is a challenge, and mandatory, lengthy addiction training courses and fellowships for primary care physicians might not be possible for everyone. However, there is potential to develop a patient-centered educational curriculum and support system that specifically addresses the stigma and social challenges that come with treating patients with addiction. This training should start early—in medical school and residency—and new physicians should enter practice with access to mentoring or peer support.

Quality metrics tied to treating patients with opioid use disorders could incentivize health systems and clinics to enroll patients into treatment programs and increase the likelihood that health systems and clinics invest resources in educational training opportunities, support staff, and psychosocial support for prescribers. These incentives could also encourage more senior providers to obtain their buprenorphine licenses, making it possible for them to then mentor the next generation of students and residents.

It has been four years since I last treated Gary. My mentors are caring for him now and have transitioned him to buprenorphine and helped him achieve sobriety. Gary's addiction treatment within a primary care setting also helped engage him in care to treat his other medical comorbidities, including his hepatitis C. I am hopeful that Gary will remain abstinent over the long term. However, I know that his addiction, much like many of the other chronic diseases I treat, might eventually relapse and remit. As I now mentor my own students and residents, Gary's story serves as a reminder of his resilience as a patient and of the need for physicians to remain supportive of their patients and of each other.

Intoxicated, Homeless, and in Need of a Place to Land

A patient with alcoholism cycles in and out of the emergency department as his providers grapple with an outdated system of care.

Otis Warren

The sun rose as the overnight shift at my emergency department (ED) came to an end. Mr. P had been with us all evening. He had arrived in an ambulance hours earlier after wandering into a home-

Volume 35, Number 11. November 2016.
Editor's Note: The patient was not identified by name to protect his identity.

less shelter, intoxicated. According to the information the ambulance staff delivered to us with Mr. P, he had been disruptive and argumentative at the shelter. According to Mr. P, the shelter staff members had been unreasonable, and he had just been minding his own business.

I performed a brief physical exam, describing in my notes a frail man, 56 years old and likely Caucasian, who had a thick gray beard and blue eyes dulled from alcohol, with subtle icterus (a yellowing of the eyes). His nose had been flattened from previous falls, and his skin was deeply sunburned, almost purple. The city's dirt had merged with his epithelial layer, giving it a rough, Velcro-like appearance.

He had unremarkable vital signs, with no new trauma and no specific medical complaints. A portable glucometer read 90 mg/dL, a normal result. He blew a 310 on the Breathalyzer—a number for which my colleagues and I had long ago forgotten the units but knew the magnitude. The textbooks would tell us at that level, Mr. P was in serious danger of alcohol poisoning, but as we already knew, he lived at this rarified level and stumbled and slurred only moderately.

From that point on, we both knew our roles. I would ignore him until the morning, and he would be given a sandwich and have the opportunity to sleep in a room with three other people in similar conditions. Before the development of our modern health care system, churches and shelters would have provided similar services when jails were not an option.

The next morning, Mr. P wanted to leave the ED—and so did I. I printed out his discharge papers, which included a list of local detoxification centers, and watched as he tossed them into the trash. As he walked out, he said a pleasant good-bye to the security guards and nurses, calling them by their first names. We knew we would see him again later that day.

The city of Providence, Rhode Island, where I work, has adopted a medical response to public intoxication like Mr. P's that involves an ambulance ride and a stay at the hospital. State laws specifically mandate this policy. If he were in another state, Mr. P might be arrested and taken to jail for the same behavior. But if he were in the same condition behind closed doors, he would be neither a patient nor a criminal. How the care for patients such as Mr. P varies from community to community exposes the paradoxical policies and philosophies behind the way alcoholism and public intoxication is treated in the United States—if it is treated at all.

Uncomplicated Intoxication

At times, I felt used by Mr. P. Last year, after we discharged him late one afternoon, he complained that we were not letting him spend the night. (Mr. P did not use our hospital's formal system for lodging complaints; instead, he preferred the expletive-laden diatribe.) I explained to him that he was no longer intoxicated, and I had to discharge him. He promised that he would return later that night, drunker, and I'd be forced to keep him until the morning. He kept his word.

Mr. P's care in our ED had been routinized to a large extent. We would use a history and physical exam to screen him for acute medical and traumatic issues. Given how frequently he came to the ED, we did not routinely document his chronic liver disease, gastritis, poorly controlled seizures, and chronic obstructive pulmonary disease, and blood work for these chronic conditions was not indicated.

Acute issues, such as when Mr. P fell, was assaulted, or had low oxygen levels, required a more thorough work-up. We had ordered hundreds of computed tomography (CT) scans of his brain (almost always with normal results) and had often admitted him to the hospital for pneumonia and other infections. But most often, his diagnosis was what we call uncomplicated intoxication, and our ED was there to ensure his safety when he could not.

Despite the challenges of caring for him, including his intoxicated outbursts, Mr. P had become beloved by most of our staff members. The nurses and technicians had spent hours dressing his wounds, caring for his hygiene, helping him to the bathroom, and listening to his stories. He could be remarkably kind when he was not too drunk.

He often asked the nurses about their families. Occasionally he gave out hugs and thanked us earnestly for caring for him. He could also be deftly funny at times. Like alcohol, his humor was warm and soothing, blunting the sharp edges of his personality and alleviating our frustrations in caring for him.

We learned from him, too. Dark humor became our own preferred elixir to quell the unpleasantness of Mr. P's inevitable health trajectory and our complicity in it. When he left the ED, we often said to each other, "We'll see him later today, unless he dies." It was a fatalistic tonic for our guilt.

On days when Mr. P didn't show up at the ED, we were concerned. He had become our neighbor, a sort of distant relative, and was subject to the same sort of worry and gossip that we would bestow upon such people. Yet for all of our worrying, we repeatedly discharged Mr. P to the street in the morning, teetering on the edge of alcohol withdrawal—a condition that could worsen and lead to tremors, hallucinations, seizures, or death. Luckily the corner liquor store opened at 7:00 a.m.

Time to Go, Mr. P

When is someone like Mr. P no longer a patient? When his blood alcohol concentration is zero, or when it reaches the legal driving limit of 0.08 percent? When he can walk steadily? When he decides to leave? What if it is cold outside? What if someone shows up and wants to take him home?

The problem was that Mr. P was intoxicated all the time; his alcohol level never reached zero while he was in our care. And no one ever showed up to take him home. In routine practice, we considered the right time to discharge him to be the "sweet spot" after his period of significant intoxication ended and before withdrawal began. If we missed this sweet spot, we might have to admit him to the hospital for alcohol withdrawal. It was a paradox and a vicious cycle: discharging Mr. P on the verge of alcohol withdrawal essentially guaranteed that he would start drinking immediately and would end up back in the ED later that day.

But what other options did we have? At 6:30 a.m., the answer was not many. In theory, there were alcohol detox programs that we could offer our patients. But these are small programs, run by community nonprofits, with a limited number of "state beds" for the uninsured. Additionally, the patient must be willing to enter the program. Mr. P had been offered detox countless times and only occasionally accepted it.

Even then, getting him into detox at the time of his discharge from the ED was nearly impossible. If he had insurance, authorization was required, and he would have to satisfy eligibility criteria. If he didn't have insurance, a bed would have to be available for someone without insurance at the very moment he needed it. Finally, most detox programs will not accept patients until their alcohol level approaches zero. Being drunk barred Mr. P from treatment for alcoholism.

I'm sure that Mr. P found it easier to go to the liquor store than to look for a detox program. For me, discharging Mr. P in this sweet spot was also the path of least resistance. Our ED is prepared to deal with critical and complex medical conditions as well as minor ones. We are equally proficient in and comfortable with treating a heart attack or an ingrown toenail. But Mr. P didn't have an acute medical condition—his social condition was the real emergency.

How complicit are we as a community in Mr. P's predicament? It was easy to blame him for his addiction and his drain on precious resources at the ED. It was harder to see how we had set up a system that took such pains to make sure that he was safe but demanded that he keep drinking to continue a lifestyle that had become comfortable for everyone.

Punitive Protection

On *The Andy Griffith Show*, Otis Campbell, the town drunk of Mayberry, would lock himself into the town jail most nights after drinking. Old Otis had come to an understanding with the sheriff that his public drinking was a crime and he needed to be locked up until he was sober. The common legal term for such a crime is "public intoxication," sometimes referred to as being drunk and disorderly—which presupposes that an intoxicated person is violating the rights of others in the community by disturbing the peace. Many states treat laws against public intoxication as public safety tools to protect an intoxicated person from harm. Much as in Mayberry, these laws are considered protective despite their punitive origins.

In 1968, the ability of the states to enforce public intoxication laws was upheld in the US Supreme Court case of *Powell v. Texas*. Mr. Powell was an alcoholic who was often intoxicated in public and frequently arrested for this offense. As a result, he had accumulated a significant number of fines that he was unable to pay. His lawyers argued that the state was punishing him for a disease. The Supreme Court disagreed and ruled that making public intoxication a crime did not violate the Eighth Amendment, which prohibits the federal government from imposing cruel and unusual punishment.

This ruling was nuanced and complicated. In its 5–4 decision, the Court found that arresting a publicly intoxicated person was a violation of the Eighth Amendment only if the person had no choice in the matter. Just six years earlier, in *Robinson v. California*, the court had ruled that drug addiction could not be punished because the addict was diseased and lacked volition in his or her drug use. In *Powell v. Texas*, the court did agree that alcoholism, like drug addiction, was a disease. But the fact that Mr. Powell had a house meant that he had chosen to drink in public. This doctrine still applies to most local responses across the country: it is not the alcoholism, but where one drinks, that is seen as the problem.

By the early 1970s, the sentiment that alcoholism is a medical condition, instead of a crime, was taking hold. Alcoholism treatment and research had come under the umbrella of the medical profession and were increasingly being funded through the newly formed National Institute on Alcohol Abuse and Alcoholism.

In 1971, the Uniform Alcoholism and Intoxication Treatment Act was drafted. This model legislation provided the legal guidelines and responses that states should adopt to address "public inebriates." It suggested that "a person who appears to be incapacitated by alcohol shall be taken into protective custody . . . and forthwith brought to an approved public treatment facility for emergency treatment." Additionally, this person "shall be examined by a licensed physician as soon as possible." The legislation urged states to set up continuities of care, which would place a publicly intoxicated person in detox instead of jail and later place the person in a longer-term sober residential treatment facility—though the specifics were to be determined by the states. Thirty-four of the 57 US jurisdictions enacted laws based on the uniform act and, as a result, were eligible for a limited amount of federal funding in the form of incentive grants to fund the programs needed for such continuities of care.

Police departments and jails were more than willing to punt homeless alcoholics back to the health care system for treatment. Soon, many states were struggling to fund the large number of detox beds they needed. At the same time, private hospitals were generally not willing to admit patients for alcoholism.

In the spirit of the uniform act, Rhode Island quickly developed a state-funded, centralized public detoxification program where patients with intoxication could be sent directly for treatment. However, after years of underfunding and allegations of mistreatment of patients, the facility closed. Large detox programs funded by states or cities across the country were facing similar problems, and detox programs were shifted to smaller nonprofit community organizations. Rhode Island's mandate that patients like Mr. P be evaluated by a physician remained, but with no centralized detoxification program and a robust modern ED, it was no surprise that Mr. P wound up with my colleagues and me.

In some states, public intoxication is still against the law. Even within a single state, enforcement can vary significantly, leading to fragmented care. In California, for instance, where public intoxication is illegal, San Diego County imposes jail sentences that increase with each violation of the law (with the option of entering an alcohol rehab program as an alternative to jail time). But San Francisco has a county-funded sobering center that serves a large number of intoxicated homeless people, and no criminal charge for public intoxication is ever filed in the city.

Social Solutions on a National Scale

A cohesive set of national policies is needed—one that recognizes not only that alcoholism is a disease but also that medical solutions alone will not solve social problems.

Across the country, some local solutions are being tried. Housing First, an assistance approach that tries to provide homeless people with permanent housing quickly and gives them supportive services as needed, holds significant promise because it recognizes that the social situation is the real emergency. Housing First would house a person like Mr. P without any requirements of sobriety. In cities where it has been studied, the program has been shown to reduce health care expenses. However, its effectiveness with people like Mr. P, who had been living on the streets for a decade and was struggling with alcoholism, has been questioned.

Diversion programs are another potential solution that treats the social situation first. Under one diversion model, if a person were picked up in a community for public intoxication, he or she would be taken to a sobering center instead of a jail or hospital. Sobering center programs range from mom-and-pop operations in church basements to sophisticated centers with nursing staffs and communications with local emergency dispatch, which coordinates the appropriate response and avoids the situation of sending a fire truck to someone sleeping on a park bench. Some of the programs are run by sheriff's departments, county health care agencies, or homeless services organizations. As diverse as the programs are, their missions are similar: to provide a safe place for people to sober up that is not a jail or a hospital. In doing so, they strive to break the cycle of chronic intoxication and provide value-based care at a reduced price.

Additionally, the confusing fog of who pays for the ED visits of patients with alcoholism has lifted. In states that expanded eligibility for Medicaid under the Affordable Care Act—including Rhode

Island—many of the previously uninsured are now covered by Medicaid. In my hospital, 70 percent of patients who had more than five visits a year for alcohol intoxication had been uninsured. Seventy percent of such patients are now covered by Medicaid, and almost none are uninsured.

One morning in early 2014, Mr. P was enrolled in Medicaid with a shaky signature before leaving the hospital. Whether or not coverage leads to communities' embracing innovative programs remains to be seen. However, Medicaid has proven flexible, and many states are using its funding to start alternative diversion programs and sobering centers to address the needs of patients like Mr. P.

In evolutionary biology, when a new ecological niche opens, diverse organisms attempt to occupy it. It is only after time has passed that the most efficient organism succeeds. While public intoxication is as old as alcohol itself, we are still looking for the best solution as various local programs across the country attempt to provide it. There have been estimates of the scope of the problem (almost 10 percent of all ED visits are related to alcohol, according to a 2012 article in the *Journal of Studies on Alcohol and Drugs*), but there are very few if any robust comparative data about solutions. The science on this topic consists of findings from individual cities and communities with differing laws and politics, leaving providers with the difficult job of identifying generalizable solutions. Moreover, US policies are remnants of the uniform act of 1971 and differ across the country. This is a national problem that has been left to local communities to solve.

Too Late

Mr. P died last autumn, having collapsed in public not long after being discharged from my ED. He was in cardiac arrest when help arrived, and he was brought to us, intoxicated and dead. It was unclear whether he had aspirated vomit into his lungs, had a heart attack, or both.

Our attempts to resuscitate him lasted for hours. In the years leading up to this moment, we had been unable to improve his life and health. Now, in cardiac arrest, Mr. P finally had a condition that my colleagues and I had been trained to treat. After multiple defibrillations, rescue medications, and chest compressions, we were able to get his heart beating again, albeit briefly. Then his pulse faded, and we started over again. As time progressed, the futility of our efforts became apparent.

Mr. P was pronounced dead in a room full of people who had cared for him nearly every day for 10 years. In an ED that regularly sees death, Mr. P's still echoes. We were his community, his friends, his family. We came to work expecting to see him, and now he had died in our hands.

As his body lay on the gurney, pale and cold, we gathered to mourn him. We lamented aloud that our final resuscitative efforts had not revived him. The truer story is that we failed him not only on the day when we could not restart his heart but also on the thousands of days when he was our patient with a beating heart and a fatal social disease.

Index